AF412704

Pediatric Airway Surgery

Advances in Oto-Rhino-Laryngology

Vol. 73

Series Editor

G. Randolph Boston, Mass.

Pediatric Airway Surgery

Volume Editors

Christopher J. Hartnick Boston, Mass.
Maynard C. Hansen Boston, Mass.
Thomas Q. Gallagher Portsmouth, Va.

130 figures, 89 in color, and 1 table, online supplementary material, 2012

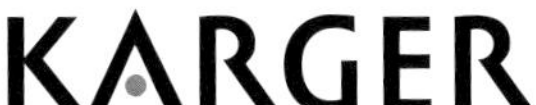

Basel · Freiburg · Paris · London · New York · New Delhi · Bangkok ·
Beijing · Tokyo · Kuala Lumpur · Singapore · Sydney

Christopher J. Hartnick
Professor, Department of Otology and Laryngology
Chief, Division of Pediatric Otolaryngology
Director, Pediatric Airway, Voice and Swallowing Center
Chief Quality Officer
Massachusetts Eye and Ear Infirmary, Harvard Medical
School
243 Charles Street
Boston, MA 02116 (USA)

Maynard C. Hansen
Massachusetts Eye and Ear Infirmary
Department of Otology and Laryngology
243 Charles Street
Boston, MA 02116 (USA)

Thomas Q. Gallagher
LCDR, MC, USN
Naval Medical Center Portsmouth
Department of Otolaryngology, Bldg 3, 4th Floor
620 John Paul Jones Circle
Portsmouth, VA 23708 (USA)

Library of Congress Cataloging-in-Publication Data

Pediatric airway surgery / volume editors, Christopher J. Hartnick, Maynard C.
Hansen, Thomas Q. Gallagher.
     p. ; cm. -- (Advances in oto-rhino-laryngology ; v. 73)
  Includes bibliographical references and index.
  ISBN 978-3-8055-9931-3 (hard cover : alk. paper) -- ISBN 978-3-8055-9932-0
(e-ISBN)
  I. Hartnick, Christopher J. II. Hansen, Maynard C. III. Gallagher, Thomas Q.
IV. Series: Advances in oto-rhino-laryngology ; v. 73.
  [DNLM: 1. Airway Obstruction--surgery. 2. Child. 3. Infant. 4.
Respiratory System--surgery. 5. Respiratory System Abnormalities--surgery.
W1 AD701 v.73 2012 / WS 280]
  617.5'40083--dc23
                                          2011051473

Bibliographic Indices. This publication is listed in bibliographic services, including Current Contents®.

© Copyright 2012 by S. Karger AG, P.O. Box, CH–4009 Basel (Switzerland)
www.karger.com
Printed in Germany on acid-free and non-aging paper (ISO 9706) by Bosch-Druck GmbH, Ergolding
ISSN 0065–3071
e-ISSN 1662–2847
ISBN 978–3–8055–9931–3
e-ISBN 978–3–8055–9932–0

Contents

Contents

 **Online supplementary material: www.karger.com/adorl073_suppl**

Preface

We conceived this book with both the training as well as the practicing surgeon in mind. The goal was to use the multi-modality possibilities provided by standard textual description in complement with both color illustrations as well as narrated high-definition video. Our premise was that our focus should be to provide a trainee or practicing surgeon with experiential pearls specific to our years of practicing pediatric airway surgery. These pearls might be in one of the following forms: specific thoughts on indications or contraindications for surgical selection, decisions on which children to operate, or choosing between a selection of possible surgeries. Other pearls might involve a close description of certain technical aspects of a given surgical procedure which we have found useful and a narrated,high-definition video demonstrating these techniques.

With the ability to use this book and view it with its accompanying free online supplementary videos, our hope is that surgeons at many levels of experience wherever they may practice (and whatever their ability to access information) will be able to access and learn from this compilation of materials. Our goal again is not an exhaustive description of the etiology, presentation, and treatment of a particular condition but rather a practical, 'surgeon's' approach to pediatric airway surgery.

Christopher J. Hartnick
Maynard C. Hansen
Thomas Q. Gallagher

Hartnick CJ, Hansen MC, Gallagher TQ (eds): Pediatric Airway Surgery. Adv Otorhinolaryngol. Basel, Karger, 2012, vol 73, pp 1–11

Laryngeal Development and Anatomy

Kedar A. Kakodkar[a] · James W. Schroeder, Jr.[b,c] · Lauren D. Holinger[b,c]

[a]Department of Otolaryngology, The University of Illinois Chicago, [b]Department of Pediatric Surgery, Children's Memorial Hospital, [c]Department of Otolaryngology, Feinberg School of Medicine, Northwestern University, Chicago, Ill., USA

Abstract

Knowledge of laryngeal and tracheobronchial development and anatomy is essential to the pediatric airway endoscopist. Normal and pathologic airway anatomy is discussed in this chapter.

Copyright © 2012 S. Karger AG, Basel

The Larynx

Certain aspects of laryngeal development and anatomy deserve particular mention. Emphasis is placed upon the infant larynx and congenital laryngeal stenosis.

Laryngeal Development
Human development is divided into the embryonic period (the first 8 weeks of gestation) and the subsequent fetal period (the last 32 weeks of gestation) [1]. The Carnegie Staging System assigns 23 stages to the embryonic period. Each stage has a characteristic feature not seen in a previous stage. Laryngeal development is first seen in stage 11 and proceeds to stage 23 and can be divided into eight phases (fig. 1).

In phase I (Carnegie stage 11), the first sign of the respiratory system is seen as an epithelial thickening along the ventral aspect of the foregut known as the respiratory primordium. In this stage, the foregut lumen is widely patent.

In phase II (Carnegie stage 12), a ventral outpouching termed the respiratory diverticulum (RD) of the foregut lumen called the primitive pharyngeal floor expands into the respiratory primordium. The primitive pharyngeal floor eventually develops in the glottic region of the adult larynx. The cephalic portion of the RD eventually develops into the infraglottic region. The RD gives rise to bilateral projections called bronchopulmonary buds that eventually develop into the lower respiratory tract.

In phase III (Carnegie stages 13 and 14), the upper foregut region and the RD migrate superiorly and the bronchopulmonary buds are drawn caudally and inferiorly [2]. As a result, the two main bronchi and carina develop. As the distance between the RD and the carina lengthens, the trachea forms. During this phase, as the trachea and esophagus lengthen, vascular compromise may cause esophageal atresia (EA), tracheoesophageal fistula (TEF), tracheal agenesis or tracheal stenosis with complete rings.

In phase IV (Carnegie stage 15), the ventral portion of the primitive laryngopharynx becomes compressed bilaterally by the developing

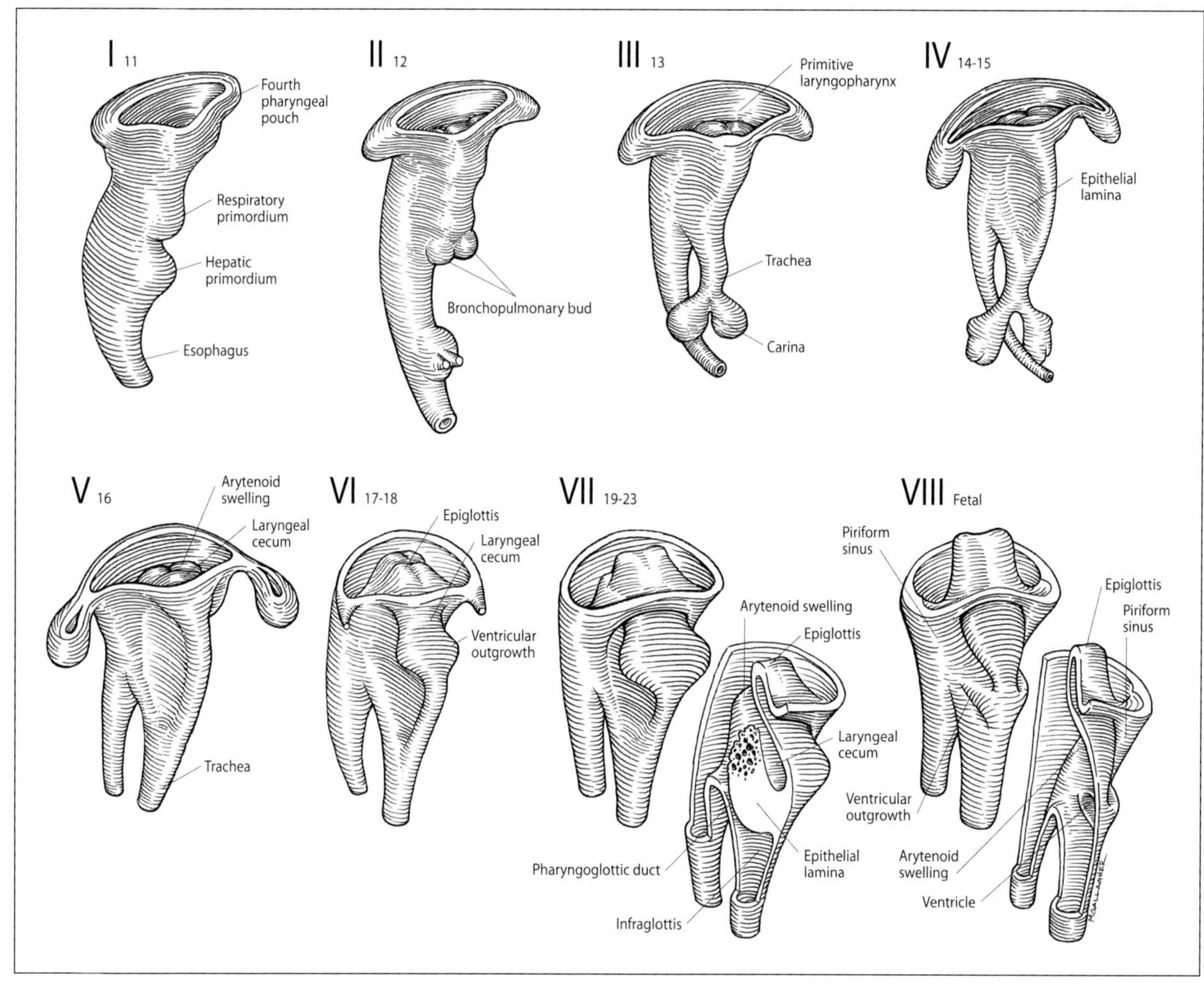

Fig. 1. Eight phases of laryngeal development.

mesoderm of the laryngeal cartilages, muscles, and the four branchial arch arteries. Eventually, the obliteration and the ventral lumen of the primitive laryngopharynx give rise to the epithelial lamina.

In phase V (Carnegie stage 16), the epithelial lamina continues to obliterate the primitive laryngopharynx in a ventral to dorsal direction leaving a narrow communication between the hypopharynx and the infraglottis. A depression called the laryngeal cecum begins to develop between the arytenoid swellings and epiglottis. The laryngeal cecum descends along the ventral aspect of the epithelial lamina giving the T-shaped entrance to the primitive laryngopharynx more definition.

In phase VI (Carnegie stages 17 and 18), the laryngeal cecum continues its caudal descent until it reaches the glottic region. In phase VII (Carnegie stages 19 and 23), the epithelial lamina begins to recanalize from a dorsocephalic to ventrocaudal direction. The last portion of the primitive laryngopharynx to recanalize is at the glottic

Kakodkar · Schroeder Jr · Holinger

level. Incomplete recanalization of the epithelial lamina can result in supraglottic and glottic webs and atresia. These atresias can be divided into three types. Type I consists of a supraglottic obstruction, absent vestibule and stenosis subglottis. Type 2 is a supraglottic obstruction that separates the primitive vestibule from the normal subglottis. In type 3, a perforated membrane partly obstructs the glottis [3].

Phase VIII of laryngeal development corresponds to the fetal period. The Carnegie staging system concludes at the end of the embryogenic period and does not apply to the fetal period. Ventral outgrowths from the lateral aspects of the laryngeal cecum give rise to the laryngeal ventricles. With complete recanalization of the epithelial lamina, a complete communication is established between the supraglottis and infraglottis.

In the fetal period, the larynx grows, becomes more defined and develops neurologic reflexes. Myenteric plexuses and ganglion cells are differentiated by 13 weeks of gestation. Fetuses begin swallowing amniotic fluid by 16 weeks' gestation. The cartilaginous vocal processes of the arytenoids as well as the ventricle and saccule are defined by this stage. Fibroelastic cartilage appears in the epiglottis in the 5th and 6th months. The corniculate cartilages develop at this time as well. During the second trimester, fetal breathing and laryngeal movement and coordination are apparent.

Laryngeal Anatomy

Cuneiform Cartilages
The cuneiform cartilages are two elastic cartilages variable in size, resting within the aryepiglottic folds anterosuperior to the arytenoid and corniculate cartilages, and without any direct articulation with the arytenoid cartilages [4] (fig. 2).

Cricoid Cartilage
The cephalad half of the cricoid cartilage is V shaped; in contrast, the caudad portion of the cricoid ring is a smooth, round circle (fig. 2). This

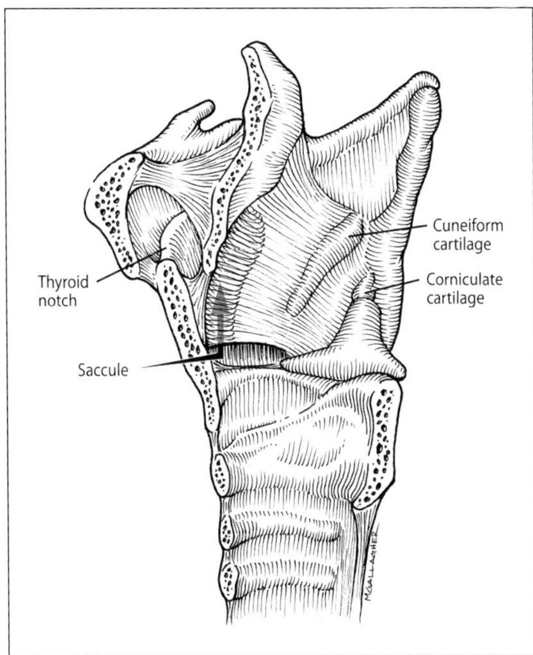

Fig. 2. The infant larynx. The saccule projects superiorly from the anterior roof of the ventricle. The hyoid bone is anterior to the thyroid notch.

produces an elliptical shape to the upper subglottic laryngeal lumen, which is somewhat more apparent in the infant than the adult.

Posterior Glottis
The anatomic boundaries defining the posterior glottis are the posterior wall of the glottis, the lateral walls of the posterior glottis, and the cartilaginous portion of the vocal folds [5]. The anterior limit of the posterior glottis is defined by the tip of the vocal process of the arytenoids.

During vocal adduction, the posterior part of the larynx closes completely, not at the glottis but at the supraglottis, resulting in the formation of a conical space in the posterior glottis that can be viewed only from below [5]. Therefore, the posterior glottis is not a commissure. The posterior glottis functions primarily for respiration and the anterior glottis for phonation.

Laryngeal Ventricle and Saccule
The laryngeal ventricle is a fusiform fossa bounded below and above the true and false vocal cords. The anterior part of the roof of the ventricle leads up into a blind pouch of mucous membrane called the *saccule*. The laryngeal saccule rises vertically between the false vocal cord and the inner surface of the thyroid cartilage [6].

The Infant Larynx

The infant larynx differs from the adult larynx in several aspects. An accurate understanding of the anatomy and histopathology of the larynx is essential in treating causes of airway obstruction, such as congenital laryngeal stenosis, as well as incomplete development resulting in posterior laryngeal cleft.

Location
The infant larynx differs from the adult larynx in a few key aspects. In the infant larynx, the inferior margin of the cricoid cartilage is at the level of the fourth cervical vertebra (C_4) and the tip of the epiglottis is at C_1. The thyroid cartilage is within the arch of the hyoid bone and slightly inferior to it (fig. 2). This laryngeal positioning allows for the epiglottis to rest posterior to the soft palate, which permits simultaneous sucking and respiration contributing to the obligate nasal breathing of the newborn [7]. As one progresses through childhood, the cricoid cartilage descends to the level of C_6 and then to the level of C_7 in the adult.

Size
At birth, the infant larynx is approximately one third the size of the adult larynx. Several structures are relatively larger in the infant larynx (see fig. 4). The vocal processes of the arytenoids comprise slightly more than half the infant glottis, whereas in the adult, they comprise approximately one seventh to one fourth the length of the glottis [5]. The cuneiform cartilages, arytenoids, and

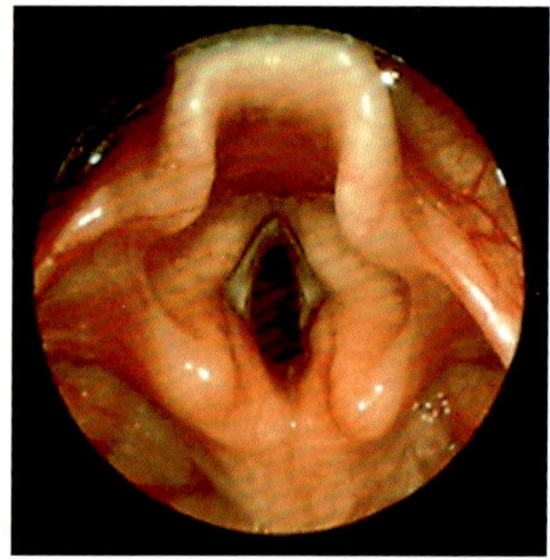

Fig. 3. Normal larynx of a 3-year-old boy. Tubular omega-shaped epiglottis is noted.

soft tissue that comprise the posterior supraglottic larynx are larger in the infant. At endoscopy, the infant larynx appears anteriorly displaced, the arytenoids are prominent and the membranous portion of the vocal fields is short. At the level of the glottis, the vocal folds are 6–8 mm in length. The posterior glottis is approximately 3–4 mm in width. The subglottic larynx has a diameter of 5–7 mm; a diameter of 4 mm represents a subglottic stenosis [8]. A 3.5-mm endotracheal tube or a size 3 bronchoscope (5 mm outside diameter) should pass through the larynx of a newborn infant without substantial resistance. The superior margin of the first tracheal arch forms a ridge often prevalent at endoscopy.

Configuration
The infant epiglottis is more narrow, posterior, and tubular or omega shaped when compared to the adult epiglottis (fig. 3). The lumen at the glottis is somewhat pentagonal in shape during inspiration. As the vocal folds taper inferiorly into the subglottic larynx, the lumen is elliptical, with the greater diameter in the anteroposterior dimension. At the inferior aspect of the cricoid cartilage, the lumen is round (fig. 4). When viewed in the coronal plane, the lumen is narrower at the top and wider at the bottom, resembling an inverted funnel. However, when viewed in the sagittal

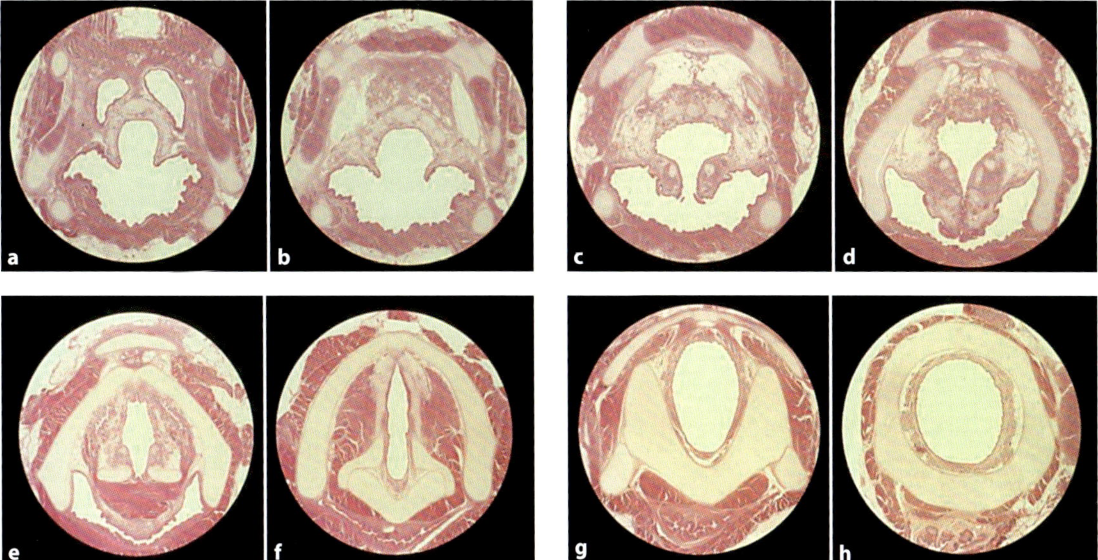

Fig. 4. Horizontal sections through the larynx of an 18-month-old child corresponding to the superior most section of the larynx at the apex of the epiglottis to the inferior most section at the inferior aspect of the cricoid cartilage (**a–h**, respectively). **a** Omega-shaped epiglottis. **b** Hyoid bone located anterior to the thyroid cartilage. **c** Saccule extends superiorly to this level. **d** Hyoid again noted to be anterior to the thyroid notch. **e** Saccule located between the false vocal fold and the inner lamina of the thyroid cartilage. **f** Superior section with V-shaped posterior cricoid cartilage. **g** Mid-section through cricoid cartilage with posterior V shape. **h** Inferior section through cricoid cartilage with a round shape. From Holinger L and others: Pediatric Laryngology and Bronchoesophagology, Lippincott-Raven, 1997.

plane, the laryngeal lumen is slightly larger superiorly at the glottic level and narrower at the inferior aspect of the cricoid cartilage. Congenital cricoid abnormalities are commonly encountered and discussed in the section below titled 'Congenital Laryngeal Stenosis' [6].

Tissue Consistency

Cartilage, muscle, and submucosal tissue are softer and more pliable in the infant larynx. Looser, less fibrous, submucosal tissue permits passive movement with respiration, and greater reaction and swelling with a more significant loss of lumen in inflammatory conditions [6].

Congenital Laryngeal Stenosis

Subglottic stenosis is one of the most common causes of airway obstruction. It can be categorized as either acquired or congenital, by clinical or anatomic characteristics, as well as by histopathology. Acquired subglottic stenosis is narrowing of the subglottic airway secondary to a traumatic or inflammatory event, most commonly endotracheal tube intubation usually in association with laryngopharyngeal reflux and infection. Subglottic stenosis is considered congenital when there is no known cause of the narrowing. Congenital subglottic stenosis, the third most common congenital laryngeal anomaly following laryngomalacia and vocal fold paralysis, is highlighted in this section [6].

With regards to the histopathologic classification, subglottic stenosis can be further categorized as either cartilaginous or soft tissue in nature. Cartilaginous subglottic stenosis can involve either a cricoid cartilage deformity or a trapped first tracheal ring. The elliptic cricoid is the most frequently diagnosed abnormal shape resulting in congenital subglottic stenosis. The ellipse pattern is due to a transverse diameter that is shorter than the anterioposterior diameter, resulting in less than normal cross-sectional area. These measurements are equal in the normal larynx. The cricoid cartilage can also assume a flattened shape with a transverse diameter greater than the anterioposterior diameter. The flattened cricoid can be associated with a trapped first tracheal ring, which involves the first tracheal ring telescoping within the cricoid cartilage causing the airway to be narrowed [9].

Upon clinical evaluation, symptoms can vary from mild stridor to severe obstruction due to the extent of the stenosis. Patients with severe obstruction may have apneic episodes, suprasternal and subcostal retractions, dyspnea, and cyanosis. Patients with congenital subglottic stenosis, particularly younger than 6 months, can also present with recurrent or persistent croup. In such patients, the underlying congenital pathology may be exacerbated by reflux events or infection, and congenital stenosis must be considered.

Evaluation of congenital laryngeal stenosis in addition to a thorough history and physical examination includes flexible fiber-optic laryngoscopy and imaging. Direct laryngoscopy and rigid bronchoscopy are vital in the assessment of congenital stenosis and also allow examination for possible synchronous airway lesions. Treatment is individualized and depends upon the nature and severity of the stenosis as well as the patient's physical condition. In general, congenital subglottic stenosis causing 50% or greater airway obstruction (Meyer-Cotton grade II or greater) may require surgical intervention, which can either be external or endoscopic approaches to cricoid expansion described in greater detail in subsequent chapters with emphasis upon surgical technique [9].

Posterior Laryngeal Cleft

The congenital posterior laryngeal cleft is a rare condition and is characterized by the incomplete development of the tracheoesophageal septum. The incidence of laryngeal cleft is approximately 1 in 10,000–20,000 live births and is more common in boys than girls, with a ratio of 5:3 [10]. A higher incidence of laryngeal cleft is reported with Pallister-Hall and Opitz-Frias syndromes [11].

Stridor, choking, cyanosis, and signs of aspiration are typical manifestations in newborns with congenital posterior laryngeal clefts. The stridor is often inspiratory but can be expiratory when associated with tracheomalacia. Other conditions that should be kept in mind when considering posterior laryngeal cleft include esophageal stricture, TEF, cricopharyngeal spasm, laryngomalacia, gastroesophageal reflux, and vocal fold paralysis.

The diagnosis of laryngeal clefts includes a high index of suspicion along with a thorough history and physical examination. Microlaryngoscopy under general anesthesia remains the gold standard in diagnosing posterior laryngeal clefts. Palpation with a probe is essential to determine the type of laryngeal cleft. In 1989, Benjamin and Inglis [10] presented a classification system in which 4 types of clefts were described: type 1 is a supraglottic interarytenoid defect that extends inferiorly no further than the level of the true vocal folds; in type 2, the cricoid lamina is partially involved with extension of the cleft below the level of the true vocal folds; type 3 is a total cricoid cleft extending inferiorly with or without further extension in the cervical trachea; type 4 extends into the posterior wall of the thoracic trachea [11].

Treatment of posterior laryngeal clefts involves initial stabilization of the infant's airway. The timing and approach for surgical repair depends on the severity of symptoms and the type of cleft present. Small clefts may be missed that often do not require surgical intervention. More significant clefts extending below the vocal folds are typically addressed via a cervical approach [6].

The Trachea and Bronchi

The anatomy of the normal tracheobronchial tree is presented in this section.

Trachea
The trachea extends from the inferior margin of the cricoid cartilage to the carina. The inferior end of the trachea is at the level of the fifth thoracic vertebra or the sternal angle. The trachea is 4 cm long in a full-term newborn infant and 11–13 cm long in an adult. The diameter of the trachea is 4–5 mm in a full-term newborn and 12–23 mm in an adult. The posterior or membranous portion of the trachea, or pars membranosa, is composed of the trachealis muscle and elastic and fibrous tissue. The ratio of cartilaginous to membranous trachea normally is 4.5:1. Variations in the tracheal cross-section diameter occur during breathing and coughing as a result of changes in head and neck position as well as intrathoracic pressure [12].

Bronchi
The trachea bifurcates at the carina, which is relatively acute in adults but less so in infants. The right main bronchus branches off at a 25° angle from the trachea, the left at a 45° [13]. Horseshoe-shaped cartilages support the main bronchi. The right main bronchus is shorter but larger in diameter than the left. The right main bronchus is straight, whereas the left often has a gentle curvature.

In normal humans, there are three lobar bronchi on the right and two on the left. Usually, there are ten segmental bronchi on the right and eight on the left. The lobar bronchi most often are constant, but there is considerable variability in the segmental bronchi. Cartilage plates support the lobar, segmental, and smaller distal bronchi [14].

The right main bronchus branches into the upper lobe bronchus and the bronchus intermedius. The upper lobe bronchus divides into anterior, posterior, and apical segments. The bronchus intermedius divides into the middle lobe and lower lobe bronchi. The middle lobe bronchus divides into medial and lateral segments. The first branch of the lower lobe bronchus is the superior segment. The remainder of the lower lobe divides into medial, anterior, lateral and posterior basal segments.

The left main bronchus divides into upper and lower lobes. The upper lobe bronchus then divides into the upper division and the lingual. The upper division has anterior and apicoposterior segments. The lingual has superior and inferior segments. The first branch of the lower lobe is the superior segment. The three basilar segments of the left lower lobe are the anteromedial, lateral, and posterior basal segments [6].

Adjacent Vascular and Cardiac Anomalies

Knowledge of adjacent anatomy and vasculature becomes particularly important when assessing etiology of external compression of the tracheobronchial tree. Tracheomalacia is the abnormal narrowing of the tracheal walls, and is classified as primary or secondary. In primary tracheomalacia, the defect is intrinsic to the trachea. No extrinsic factors cause compression or distortion, and the cartilage-to-membranous trachea ratio may be 3 to 1, or even 2 to 1. The flattened posterior membranous trachea collapses forward during expiration (and more so with coughing), often touching the anterior wall. In secondary tracheomalacia, other factors are related to the pathology. Similarly, bronchomalacia is the abnormal narrowing of the bronchial walls, which can also be secondary to adjacent pathology. In particular, certain types of vascular and cardiac abnormalities are noted to cause specific presenting symptoms and characteristic endoscopic findings and are discussed below.

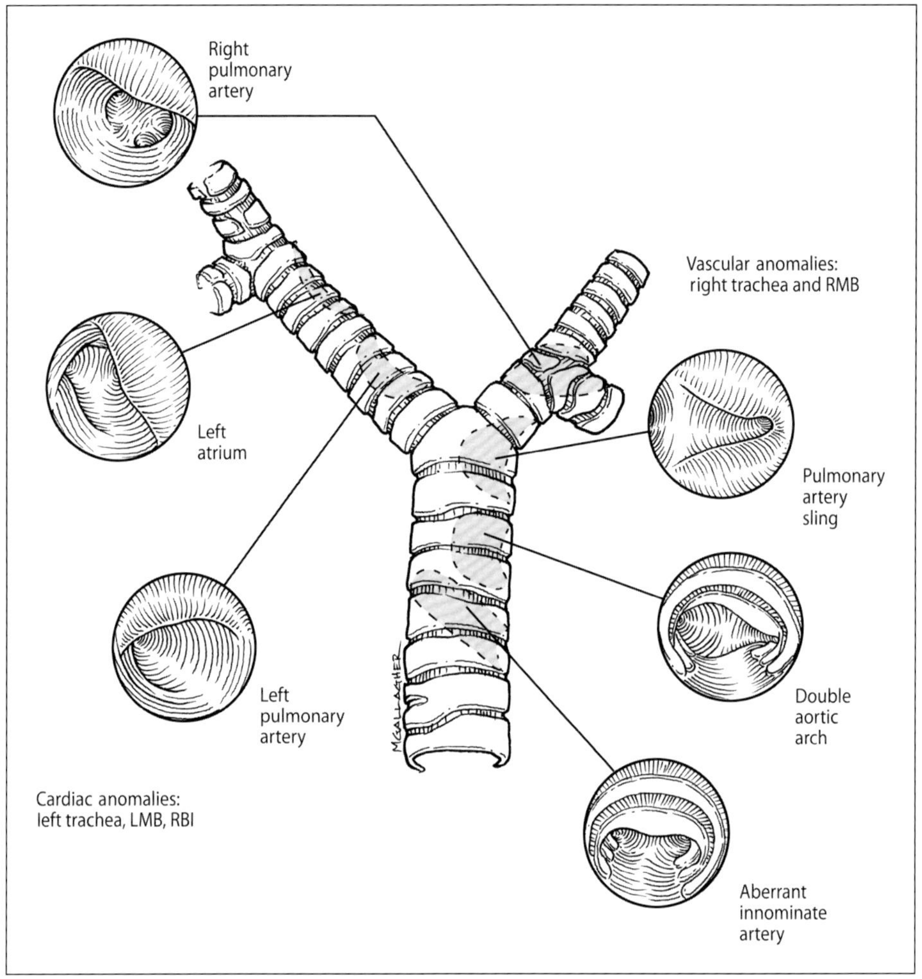

Fig. 5. Endoscopic depiction of the tracheobronchial tree and typical findings secondary to adjacent vascular pathology and cardiovascular disease.

Aberrant Innominate Artery

An aberrant innominate artery may cause compression of the trachea seen on endoscopy as compression of the right anterolateral wall of the upper trachea, giving the lumen a triangular shape (fig. 5). Lifting the tip of the bronchoscope against the pulsatile artery diminishes the right brachial pulse. This compression can lead to a variety of presenting symptoms, including a croupy or barky cough, wheezing, expiratory stridor, or apneic episodes. The differential diagnosis to be considered includes central apnea, gastroesophageal reflux with apnea, and other causes of apparent life-threatening events [6].

Patients with severe obstruction and subsequent life-threatening episodes, recurrent pneumonia due to ineffective clearance of secretions, and progressive obstruction may warrant suspension of the innominate artery and aorta to the posterior surface of the sternum (innominate arteriopexy). Yet, the majority of patients with an aberrant innominate artery resulting in extrinsic airway compression do not require surgical intervention due to its self-limiting nature.

Double Aortic Arch
The double aortic arch is a relatively rare congenital anomaly in which two aortic arches form a complete vascular ring that encircles the trachea and esophagus, forming a complete ring (fig. 5). Most commonly, there is a dominant right arch posterior and a hypoplastic left arch anterior to the trachea and esophagus. The two arches subsequently join the descending aorta, which is usually on the left side.

Symptoms related to this anomaly are due to the compression of the trachea and/or the esophagus and usually begin at birth. Diagnosis can often be suspected or made by radiograph, barium esophagram, or echocardiography. Computer tomography or magnetic resonance imaging are more specific and note the anatomic relationship of the aortic arches to the trachea and esophagus. This aids the cardiovascular surgeon in planning surgical division of the ring. Many patients experience almost immediate postoperative resolution of obstructive symptoms, whereas in some it takes 1–2 years for respiratory symptoms to improve [6].

Pulmonary Artery Sling
The pulmonary artery (PA) sling is associated with an absent left PA and is, instead, associated with an aberrant left PA arising from the right PA. Upon endoscopy, this vascular anomaly may cause compression of the right main bronchus, which may have a slit-like lumen and subsequently courses between the trachea and esophagus (fig. 5). The lower trachea is narrowed from the right side. Treatment includes surgery to divide and reimplant the artery, improving obstructive symptoms [15].

Congenital Cardiac Defects
Pulmonary hypertension secondary to a left-to-right shunt can lead to enlargement of the pulmonary arteries and subsequent compression of the left main bronchus (fig. 5). The left main bronchus normally traverses the superior aspect of the left atrium and left pulmonary veins, also passing adjacent to the pulmonary arteries. Patients with ventral septal defects or patent ductus arteriosus may have such compression secondary to left-to-right shunt and resulting pulmonary hypertension [15].

Symptoms depend upon the severity of airway obstruction and may include wheezing, recurrent pneumonia, atelectasis, or lobar emphysema. Severe cases may include ventilator dependence due to high mean airway pressures needed to overcome compressed airways. Bronchoscopy may yield left-sided bronchial compression. Computed tomography of the chest with contrast, magnetic resonance imaging, or cardiac catheterization may reveal the underlying pathology. Treatment is targeted towards relief of pulmonary hypertension and subsequent airway compression. PA plication or arteriopexy are rarely indicated [16].

Tracheoesophageal Fistula and Esophageal Atresia

A TEF is an abnormal connection between the esophagus and the trachea. Congenital EA results in two blind-ended pouches, an upper and a lower, which may or may not communicate with the tracheobronchial tree resulting in a TEF. Presenting symptoms include feeding and/or respiratory difficulties as well as persistent aspiration. TEF and EA occur in approximately 1 in 3,000–5,000 births. The five forms of EA and TEF are illustrated in figure 6. Treatment is surgical and involves primary extrapleural repair of EA with division and oversewing of the distal fistula. Postsurgical complications include tracheomalacia, esophageal stricture, recurrent fistula, and gastroesophageal reflux. The prognosis of surgical intervention is good, but respiratory complications may be severe [17].

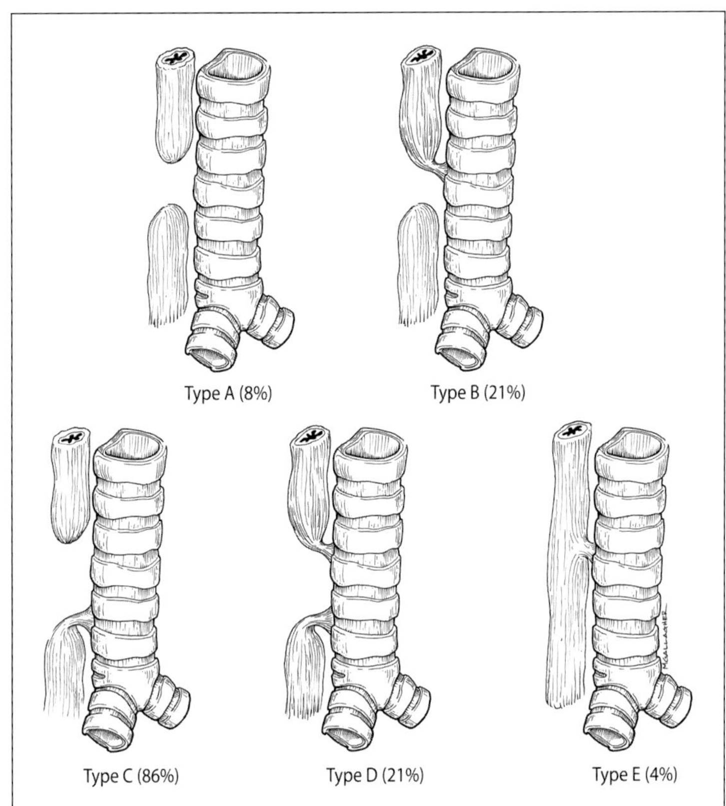

Fig. 6. Five types of EA and tracheoesophageal atresia. Type C is the most common.

Conclusions

The pediatric airway endoscopist must be well versed in the normal and pathologic anatomic and developmental variations. Knowledge of key structural features involving the larynx, trachea and bronchi is essential in understanding the diagnosis and treatment of congenital laryngeal stenosis, posterior laryngeal cleft, external compression secondary to adjacent vascular and cardiac anomalies, as well as EA and TEF.

References

1 Henick DH: Three dimensional analysis of murine laryngeal development. Ann Otol Rhinol Laryngol Suppl 1993;159:3–24.

2 O'Rahilly R, Müller F: Chevalier Jackson lecture. Respiratory and alimentary relations in staged human embryos. New embryological data and congenital anomalies. Ann Otol Rhinol Laryngol 1984:93:421–429.

3 Zaw-Tun HI: Development of congenital laryngeal atresias and cleft. Ann Otol Rhinol Laryngol 1988;97:353.

4 Bosma JF: Anatomy of the Infant Head. Baltimore, The John Hopkins University Press, 1985.

5 Hirano M, Kurita S, Kiyokawa K, Sato K: Posterior glottis. Morphological study in excised human larynges. Ann Otol Rhino Laryngol 1986;95:576–581.

6 Holinger LD: Pediatric Laryngology & Bronchoesophagology. Philadelphia, Lippincott Raven, 1997.

7 Holinger PH, Johnson KC, Schiller F: Congenital anomalies of the larynx. Ann Otol Rhino Laryngol 1954;63:581–606.

8 Schild JA: Relationship of laryngeal dimensions to body size and gestational age in premature, neonates and small infants. Laryngoscope 1984;94:1284–1292.

9 Schroeder JW, Holinger LD: Congenital laryngeal stenosis. Otol Clin North Am 2008;41:865–875.
10 Benjamin B, Inglis A: Minor congenital laryngeal clefts: diagnosis and classification. Ann Otol Rhinol Laryngol 1989;98:417–420.
11 William PL, Warwick R (eds): Gray's Anatomy, ed 36. Philadelphia, WB Saunders, 1980, p 1246.
12 Hollinshead WH, Rosse C: Textbook of Anatomy, ed 4. Philadelphia, Harper & Row, 1985, p 494.
13 Williams PL, Warwick R (eds): Gray's Anatomy, ed 36. Philadelphia, WB Saunders, 1980, p 1257.
14 Landing BH, Dixon LG: Congenital malformations and genetic disorders of the respiratory tract. Am Rev Respir Dis 1979;120:151–185.
15 Holinger PH: Congenital anomalies of the tracheobronchial tree. Postgrad Med 1964;26:454–462.
16 Benjamin B, Pham T: Diagnosis of H-type tracheoesophageal fistula. J Pediatr Surg 1991;26:667–671.
17 Benjamin B: Endoscopy in esophageal atresia and tracheoesophageal fistula. Ann Otol Rhinol Laryngol 1981;90:376.

James W. Schroeder, Jr.
Children's Memorial Hospital
Department of Pediatric Surgery
Chicago, IL 60614 (USA)
E-Mail jschroeder@childrensmemorial.org

Hartnick CJ, Hansen MC, Gallagher TQ (eds): Pediatric Airway Surgery. Adv Otorhinolaryngol. Basel, Karger, 2012, vol 73, pp 12–18

Flexible Bronchoscopy

Lael M. Yonker[a] · M. Shannon Fracchia[a,b]

[a]Pediatric Pulmonary Department, Massachusetts General Hospital, and [b]Massachusetts Eye and Ear Infirmary, Pediatric Airway Clinic, Boston, Mass., USA

Abstract

Flexible bronchoscopy is an important procedure for evaluating the pediatric airway, allowing a dynamic view from the trachea through the lower bronchi. The flexible bronchoscope offers greater maneuverability than the rigid bronchoscope and may be done in conjunction with other procedures, such as bronchoalveolar lavage, transbronchial biopsy, endobronchial ultrasound, electrocautery or laser treatments. Common indications for flexible bronchoscopy include recurrent croup or pneumonia, aspiration, foreign body and chronic cough. Although bronchospasm, transient fever, infection and pneumothorax are rare complications of flexible bronchoscopy, these risks are minimized with careful technique and an ongoing dialogue with the anesthesiologist. Flexible bronchoscopy is an important tool in the diagnosis, monitoring and therapy of certain pulmonary diseases and should be considered in the management of carefully selected pediatric patients.

Flexible bronchoscopy is an important modality used to examine the airway, offering diagnostic information regarding the upper and lower airway structures, in addition to providing means for obtaining samples of airway tissue and bronchoalveolar fluid. Made of fiber-optic rods or a distal imaging device with digital transmission, a bronchoscope comes in a variety of sizes for a wide age range, and is generally equipped with a separate suction/instrument channel. Flexible bronchoscopy can be performed independently or in conjunction with rigid bronchoscopy, and is often useful in evaluation of recurrent croup, atypical cough, hemoptysis or wheeze.

One of the greatest benefits of flexible bronchoscopy is that it offers a dynamic view of the airway, which is essential to diagnose tracheo- or bronchomalacia or compression of the airway. The smaller size of the flexible bronchoscope permits a view of the lower airways, which would not be possible with the larger rigid bronchoscope. This maneuverability allows for assessment of suspected foreign body or lower airway obstruction.

Additionally, there are several procedures done through flexible bronchoscopy which often aid in diagnosis or monitoring of an illness. The most commonly performed procedure done in conjunction with flexible bronchoscopy is bronchoalveolar lavage which not only allows removal of mucous plugs or debris but also provides sampling from the lower airways which may be sent for microbacterial and cytological analysis. Transbronchial or endobronchial biopsies may also be performed and are less invasive alternatives to an open lung biopsy. Endobronchial ultrasound, electrocautery and laser treatments may also be performed via flexible bronchoscope, and as technology grows, flexible bronchoscopy will continue to offer invaluable assistance in the evaluation and management of airway lesions.

Indications

- Recurrent croup
- Recurrent pneumonia
- Aspiration
- Foreign body
- Cough
- Suspected airway compression
- Wheezing
- Hemoptysis
- Pulmonary alveolar proteinosis (rare condition)

Contraindications

- Cardiovascular instability
- Bleeding diathesis
- Severe bronchospasm
- Hypoxemia

Complications

- Bronchospasm
- Transient fever
- Infection
- Pneumothorax

Anesthesia Considerations

When performing a bronchoscopy on a pediatric patient, it is extremely important to have an ongoing dialogue with the anesthesiologist regarding the patient's respiratory status. Since instrumenting the airway can be irritating to the tracheobronchial tree and pediatric patients have lower pulmonary reserve than adult patients, the pulmonologist may have to remove the bronchoscope from the airway intermittently to allow the anesthesiologist to recover adequate ventilation. The size of the bronchoscope may also have implications on the respiratory status of the pediatric patient: even when an age-appropriate-sized bronchoscope is used, it may still occlude the upper airway, particularly if the airway is maintained with an endotracheal tube. For this reason, using an laryngeal mask airway (LMA) when performing a bronchoscopy, if possible, may offer better ventilatory control. Vocal cord spasm and bronchospasm are often triggered by contact with the bronchoscope and are minimized by instillation of local anesthetic (0.5–1 ml of 2% lidocaine) at the level of the vocal cords and the carina.

Bronchoscopy Set-Up

The set-up is as depicted in figures 1 and 2:
- Bronchoscope
- Bronchofiberscope, hybrid bronchofibervideoscope or bronchovideoscopes of age-/size-appropriate diameter
- Tower: light source, video system center/monitor (recording, keyboard, printer)
- Lubricant jelly
- Sterile gauze 4 × 4s
- Swivel adaptor for LMA/endotracheal tube
- 2% lidocaine without preservative
- 5-ml syringe for inserting lidocaine
- Sterile 0.9% normal saline for lavage
- 10- or 20-ml syringes for instillation of 0.5–1cc/kg normal saline for bronchoalveolar lavage
- Sputum traps
- Suction
- Gloves

Additional Equipment
- Endobronchial forceps
- Cytology brushes
- Transbronchial biopsy forceps and C-arm X-ray machine for guidance radiographic imaging
- Sterile container for brushings/biopsies

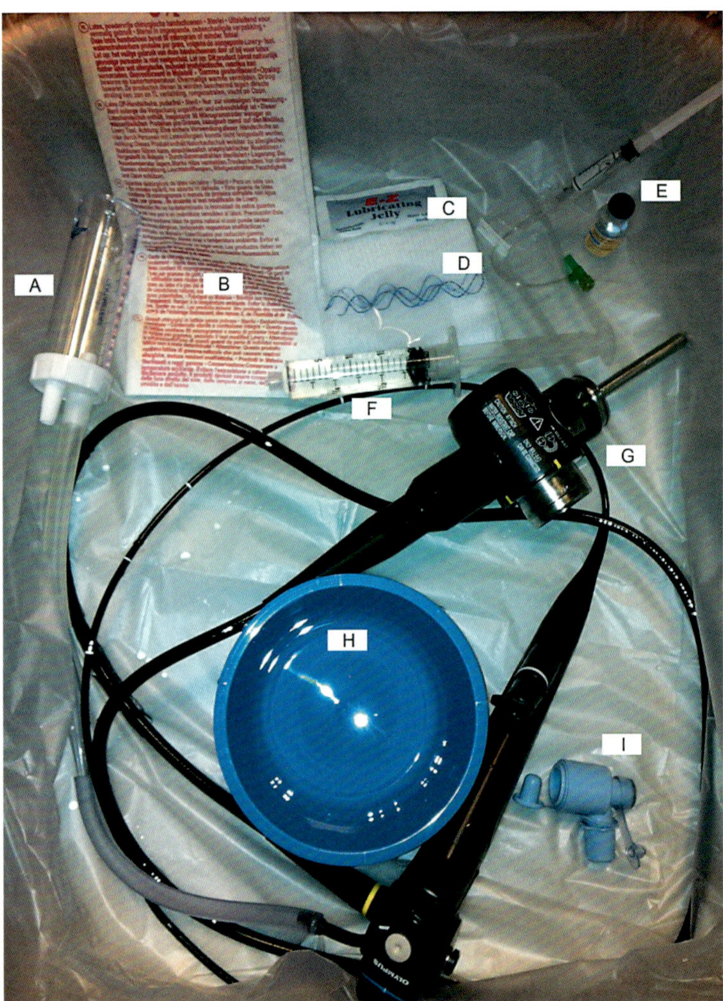

Fig. 1. Bronchoscopy set up. A: Suction trap attached to bronchoscopy and suction. Care must be taken to hold the suction trap vertically during the procedure as not to lose the content to the wall suction. Having extension tubing as shown allows the suction trap to hang in a more vertical position. B: Gloves. C: Lubricating jelly. D: Sterile gauze 4 × 4s with some dispensed lubricating jelly. E: 2% lidocaine, draw up into a 3-ml syringe with tubing and male adaptor to allow instillation into the bronchoscope. F: 20-ml syringe with normal saline. After the lidocaine has been dispensed, the adaptor may be transferred to the saline for dispense. G: Bronchoscope. H: Sterile bowl filled with normal saline which may be used judiciously to help clear the bronchoscope of plugs once the bronchoscope is removed from the airway. Oversuctioning of saline will dilute the sample. I: Swivel adaptor for LMA/endotracheal tube.

- Aspiration needles
- Grasping forceps
- Balloon catheters
- Ultrasonic probes
- Laser and electrosurgical attachments

Procedures

- Bronchoalveolar lavage:
- Cell count
- Microbiology/culture
- Lipid-laden macrophages
- Hemosiderin-laden macrophages
- Cytology
- Flow cytometry
- Brush biopsy
- Endobronchial biopsy
- Transbronchial biopsy
- Endobronchial ultrasound
- Segmental bronchography, brochoscopic treatment of airway and pulmonary bleeding, endoscopy-assisted tracheal intubation, bronchial dilation, stent placement

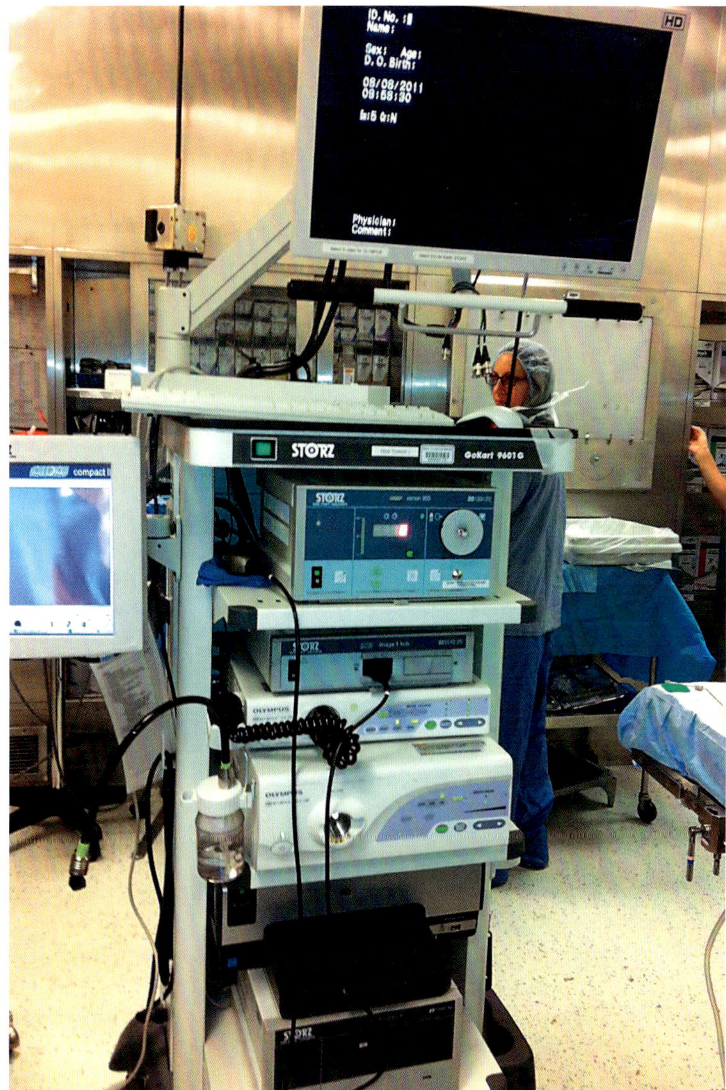

Fig. 2. Bronchoscope tower. The bronchoscope tower is comprised of video monitor, keyboard and mouse, light source, video processor, recording equipment and printer.

Common Findings

- Normal anatomy (online suppl. video 1)
- Video 1: Overview of flexible bronchoscopy: bronchomalacia of left main bronchus, otherwise normal anatomy. This video describes the procedure of flexible bronchoscopy while progressing through normal anatomic landmarks: trachea, carina, right upper lobe, right middle lobe, right basal segments of the right lower lobe, left upper lobe , lingula and the left basal segments of the left lower lobe in addition to visualizing each lobe's segmental branches. Bronchoalveolar lavage is also demonstrated. This patient's anatomy is notable for bronchomalacia, or collapse, of the left main bronchus.
- Tracheomalacia: weakness or floppiness of the tracheal wall causing the trachea to be more

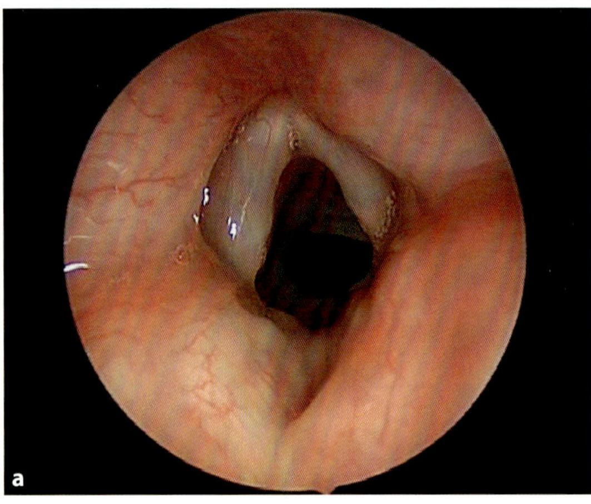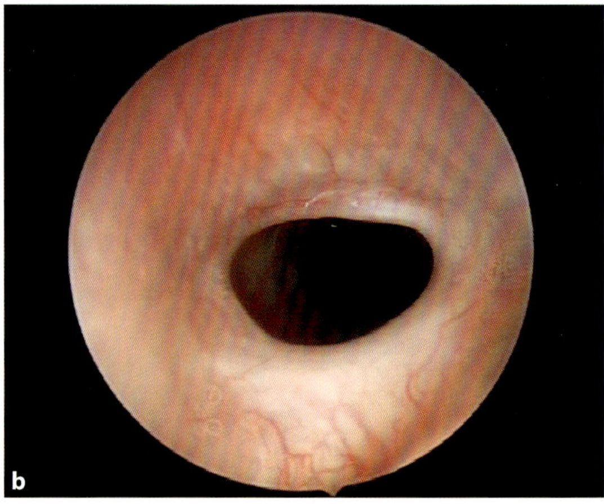

Fig. 3. Tracheal stenosis. Circumferential narrowing of the tracheal lumen is viewed from above the vocal cords (**a**) and a close-up picture (**b**).

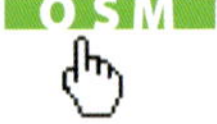

susceptible to collapse, which is not as easily appreciated with a rigid bronchoscope (online suppl. video 2)

– Video 2: tracheomalacia and tracheo-esophageal fistula (TEF). As the bronchoscope is passed through the trachea, severe inward collapse of the tracheal wall is present. This case was severe enough to warrant tracheostomy tube placement, visible through the anterior wall of the mid-/upper trachea. As the bronchoscope is passed more distally through the trachea, a small defect is seen in the posterior tracheal wall, just above the level of the carina, representing a previously closed H-type TEF. Of note, although tracheomalacia is a relatively common finding in children with persistent cough or noisy breathing, TEF/esophageal atresia is a rare finding, reported as occurring in 1 in every 5,000 births. An H-type TEF accounts for 4–5% of these cases [1]. In cases of TEF, however, 75% of patients will have some degree of tracheomalacia [2].

- Bronchomalacia: weakness of a segment of bronchus causing collapse or compression and interferes with bronchociliary clearance (online suppl. video 1)

- Stenosis: fixed reduction in airway lumen due to abnormal development or secondary to endobronchial injury and inflammation (fig. 3)
- Compression: fixed narrowing of the trachea or bronchus, which may be pulsatile indicating arterial compression
- Bronchus suis (translated as pig bronchus, also known as tracheal bronchus): normal anatomic variant defined as having the right upper lobe bronchus diverge off the trachea, above the level of the carina, rather than from the right main bronchus (online suppl. video 3; fig. 4)
– Video 3: bronchus suis and tracheal hemangioma. Passing through the trachea, an outpouching is seen off the right side of the tracheal wall which is consistent with a bronchus suis. Adjacent to the bronchus suis is a raised vascular lesion representing an airway hemangioma. There is no association with airway hemangiomas and a bronchus suis.
- Hemangiomas: a vascular lesion which may compress or obstruct the airway, usually growing in size over the first year of life then receding. Multiple facial hemangiomas, particularly over the beard region, is a risk factor for having a hemangioma within the airway (online suppl. video 3).

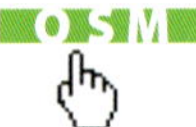

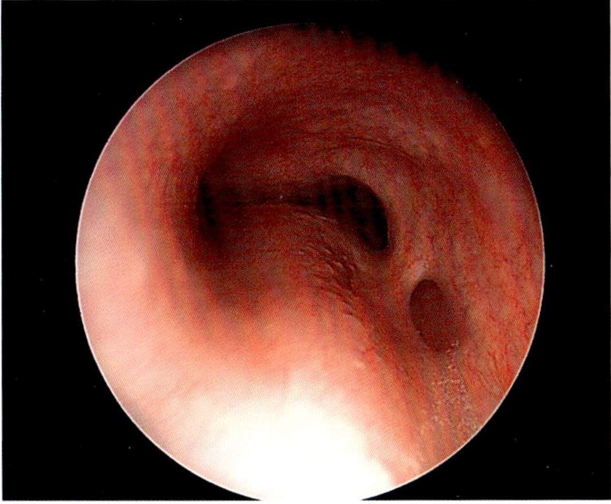

Fig. 4. Bronchus suis (pig bronchus, also referred to as tracheal bronchus). A normal anatomic variant in 0.1% of the population. Of note, there is also increased nodularity of the tracheal mucosa suggesting inflammation.

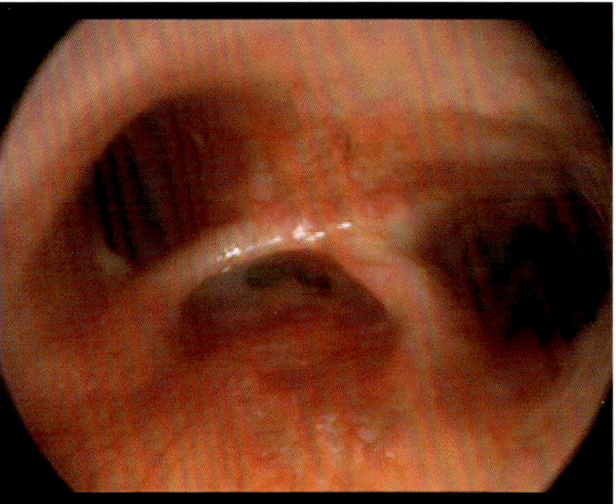

Fig. 5. H-type TEF. Although most TEFs are diagnosed in the newborn period as a result of esophageal atresia, the H-type TEF, shown here as an out-pouching in the distal posterior segment of the posterior tracheal wall connecting the trachea to the esophagus is the most common cause of TEF diagnosed in older children. This TEF is status post repair 3 years ago, but the residual defect in the tracheal wall remains, although now closed off to the esophagus.

- TEF: although there are several types of TEFs typically diagnosed in the newborn period due to esophageal atresia, the one that is most often diagnosed in older children is the H-type TEF. In the case of the H-type TEF, a small airway defect is seen typically along the base of the posterior wall of the trachea, connecting the airway with the patent esophagus (online suppl. video 2; fig. 5).
- Abnormal mucosa: the mucosa may be inflamed, edematous with loss of clarity of cartilaginous rings or nodular
- Secretions: secretions may be seen in any part of the airway and may be thin and clear or frothy, or thick, purulent and tenacious, usually making them more difficult to extract through the channels of the bronchoscope
- Foreign bodies

Pearls

- Benefits of flexible bronchoscopy compared to rigid bronchoscopy include its smaller size, dynamic view, increased maneuverability, and ability to visualize lower airways
- Certain procedures such as bronchoalveolar lavage and transbronchial biopsy may be performed in conjuction with flexible bronchoscopy
- Common indications include recurrent croup, pneumonia, aspiration, suspicion of foreign body, chronic cough or wheeze
- Common findings include tracheomalacia, bronchomalacia, stenosis, edematous or nodular mucosa
- Risks of flexible bronchoscopy include bronchospasm, transient fever, infection, pneumothorax
- An ongoing dialogue with the anesthesiologist is important to minimize bronchospasm and avoid complications

For similar information on pediatric flexible bronchoscopy we recommend the book 'Paediatric Bronchoscopy', Eds. Prifits et al. [4].

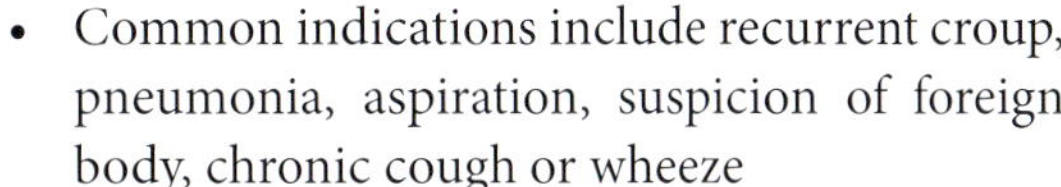

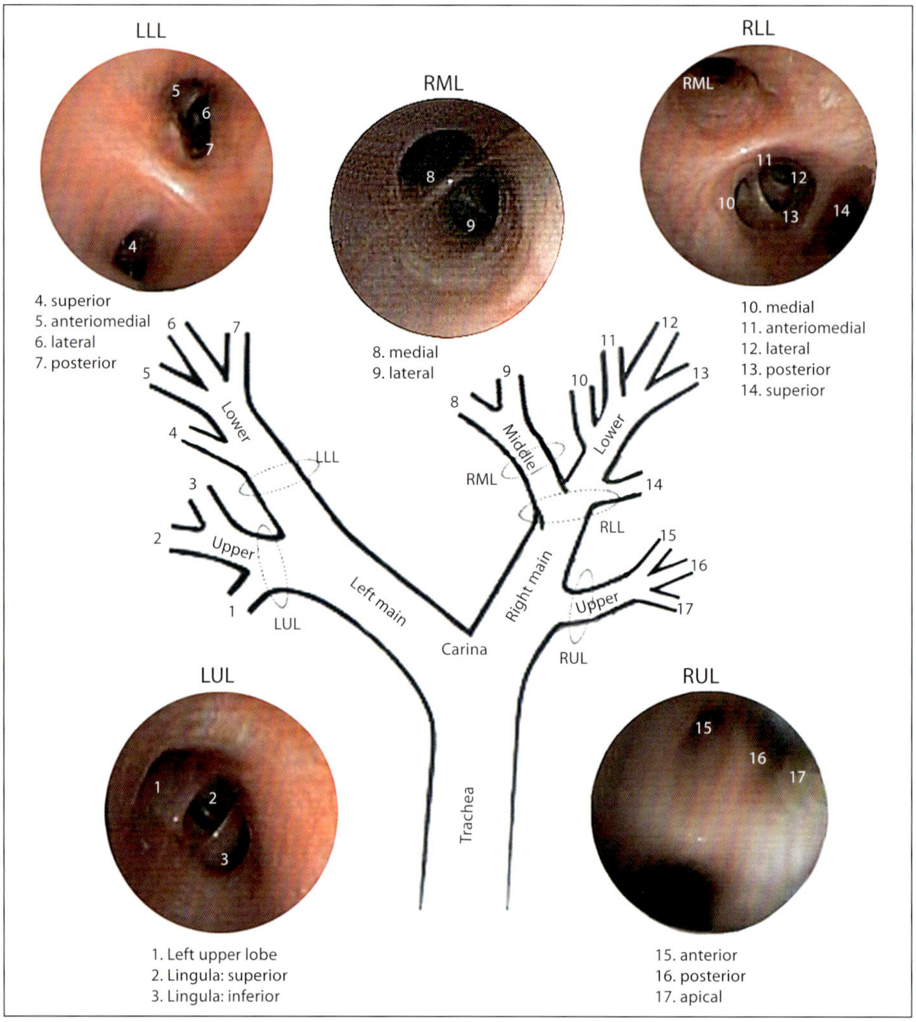

Fig. 6. Normal pulmonary anatomy with bronchoscopic views of lower airways. LUL = Left upper lobe; LLL = left lower lobe; RML = right middle lobe; RLL = right lower lobe; RUL = Right upper lobe. Created by Alexis Cook and Matthew Brudner.

References

1 Achildi O, Grewal H: Congenital anomalies of the esophagus. Otolaryngol Clin North Am 2007;40:219–244.
2 Spitz L: Esophageal atresia and tracheoesophageal fistula in children. Curr Opin Pediatr 1993;5:347–352.
3 Webb WR, Higgins CB: Thoracic Imaging: Pulmonary and Cardiovascular Radiology, North American Edition, ed 2. Philadelphia, Wolters Kluwer/Lippincott Williams & Wilkins, 2011.
4 Priftis KN, Anthracopoulos MB, Eber E, Koumbourlis AC, Wood RE, ed. Paediatric Bronchoscopy, in Bollinger CT, ed, Progress in Respiratory Research. vol 38. Basel, Karger, 2010.

Lael M. Yonker, MD
Massachusetts General Hospital
Pediatric Pulmonary Department
275 Cambridge Street
Boston, MA 02114 (USA)
E-Mail lyonker@partners.org

Hartnick CJ, Hansen MC, Gallagher TQ (eds): Pediatric Airway Surgery. Adv Otorhinolaryngol. Basel, Karger, 2012, vol 73, pp 19–25

Direct Laryngoscopy and Rigid Bronchoscopy

Thomas Q. Gallagher[a] · Christopher J. Hartnick[b]

[a]LCDR, MC, USN, Department of Otolaryngology, Naval Medical Center Portsmouth, Portsmouth, Va.,
[b]Department of Otology and Laryngology, Massachusetts Eye & Ear Infirmary, Boston, Mass., USA

Abstract

Laryngoscopy and rigid bronchoscopy represent a necessary tool in the otolaryngologist's arsenal. The advancement in designing smaller and more versatile laryngeal equipment and fiber-optic telescopes as well as the increasingly higher resolution of still and video imagery have allowed otolaryngologists to better diagnose and treat many airway lesions. This chapter describes the basic equipment necessary as well step-by-step description of the technique to perform rigid airway endoscopy.

Endoscopy has become an invaluable tool to the aerodigestive surgeon. Since its early beginnings with German physician Philipp Bozzini (1773–1809) and his 'Lichtleiter' ('light guide' – a double cannula with internal mirror device using candle light to allow inspection of the larynx), endoscopists have pushed the envelope to better see and understand the aerodigestive tract [1]. Soon others followed: Manuel Garcia (1805–1906) pioneered autolaryngoscopy; Dr. Alfred Kirsten (1895)

The views expressed in this article are those of the authors and do not necessarily reflect the official policy or position of the Department of the Navy, Department of Defense, or the United States Government.

Thomas Q. Gallagher is a military service member. This work was prepared as part of his official duties. Title 17 .S.C. 105 provides that 'Copyright protection under this title is not available for any work of the United States Government.' Title 17 U.S.C. 101 defines a United States Government work as a work prepared by a military service member or employee of the United States Government as part of that person's official duties.

moved away from indirect mirror laryngoscopy with direct visualization of the larynx; Dr. Gustav Killian (1911, 'Father of Bronchoscopy'), with the advent of suspension, made bimanual manipulation of the larynx possible; from this point in Philadelphia, Dr. Chevalier Jackson ('Father of American Bronchoesophagology') began his practice and would then train Dr. Paul Holinger, father and mentor of Dr. Lauren Holinger.

In the 1930s and 1940s, Dr. P. Holinger along with photographic engineers James and Joseph Brubaker successfully developed the first hand-held endoscopic camera. In 1941, they produced the first high-quality film of the bronchial tree and then the first high quality photos of the larynx. Please note this list of notable physicians does not include all those (physician and scientists) that pioneered the technology of endoscopy, names like Nitze, von Mikulicz, Fourestier, Lamm, van Heel and Hopkins. Since then, the evolution of technology and innovation has produced even smaller and more versatile instruments, telescopes and cameras allowing endoscopists to better evaluate, diagnose and treat pediatric aerodigestive disorders.

Both flexible and rigid bronchoscopy are necessary procedures in order to fully evaluate the pediatric airway. Advantages of rigid bronchoscopy include the ability to ventilate while performing bronchoscopy, which is helpful for patients with poor pulmonary reserve, as well as superior optics and resolution. Flexible bronchoscopy allows for visualization and access to the smaller airways and the ability to perform diagnostic procedures (i.e. bronchoalveolar lavage). Also of significance is the evaluation of tracheo- and bronchomalacia. Flexible bronchoscopy is superior to rigid bronchoscopy in the evaluation of malacia by giving the endoscopist a dynamic view of the airway during respiration. Rigid bronchoscopy artifactually stents the airway open during the procedure giving the endoscopist a false sense of airway patency.

Performing both flexible and rigid bronchoscopy is complementary adding the collective benefits together to gain a better understanding of the pathology. Additionally, with the addition of a pulmonologist to the 'team', broader differentials can be entertained to achieve the correct diagnosis. In this chapter, the authors will describe their technique for evaluation of the pediatric larynx, trachea, and bronchi to include some instruments and pearls necessary for success.

Relevant Anatomy

For relevant anatomy, see the Laryngeal Development and Anatomy chapter.

Indications

- SPECSR acronym [2]
- Severity: subjective impression from parents/ guardian
- Progression: the lesion has become larger over time
- Eating: feeding difficulties, concern for aspiration, weight loss
- Cyanotic episodes: Child turning blue or apparent life-threatening events
- Sleep: obstructive symptoms while sleeping (i.e. retractions)

- Radiology: findings on radiographs suggestive of an airway lesion.
- Concerning findings on office-based flexible fiber-optic laryngoscopy

Contraindications

Significant subglottic stenosis where any instrumentation of the airway at the point of the stenosis may cause imminent respiratory compromise

Anesthesia Considerations

- Open and ongoing dialogue with the anesthesiologist
- The table and the patient's airway are turned over to the endoscopist during the procedure. Allowing the anesthesia provider to see the video display can help them understand the nuances of the case so they can maintain the correct plane of anesthesia.
- If a ventilating bronchoscope is utilized, switching the anesthesia circuit will be necessary during the case
- A one-time dose of dexamethasone 0.5 mg/kg up to 10 mg

Preparation

- Equipment needed:
- Straight blade laryngoscope (Miller or Parsons)
- The straight blade laryngoscopes allow safe and straight passage of the telescope or rigid bronchoscope through the laryngeal inlet without local tissue damage or bending of the telescope
- Basic pediatric rigid bronchoscopy set (fig. 1)
- Lindholm vocal cord and false cord retractor (Karl Storz, Germany; fig. 2)

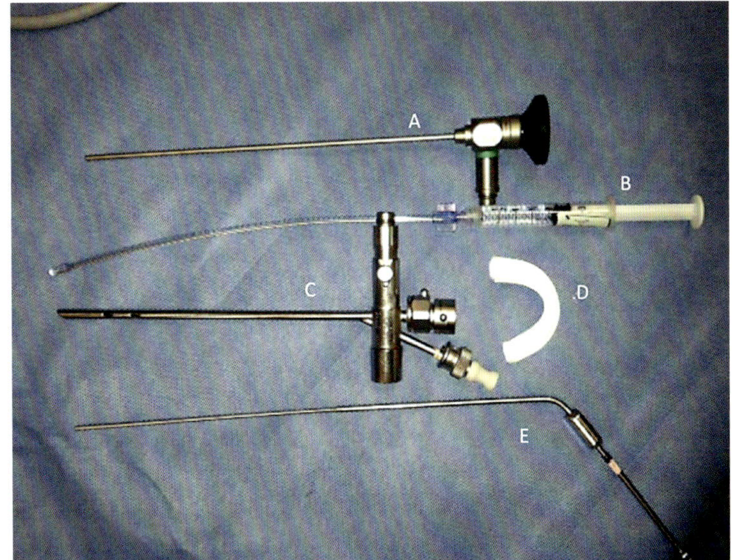

Fig. 1. Pediatric direct laryngoscopy and bronchoscopy equipment. A: 0° 4 mm × 18 cm Hopkins rod-lens telescope; B: 4% lidocaine with atomizer; C: Ventilating bronchoscope; D: Tooth guard; E: Laryngeal microsuction with thumb control.

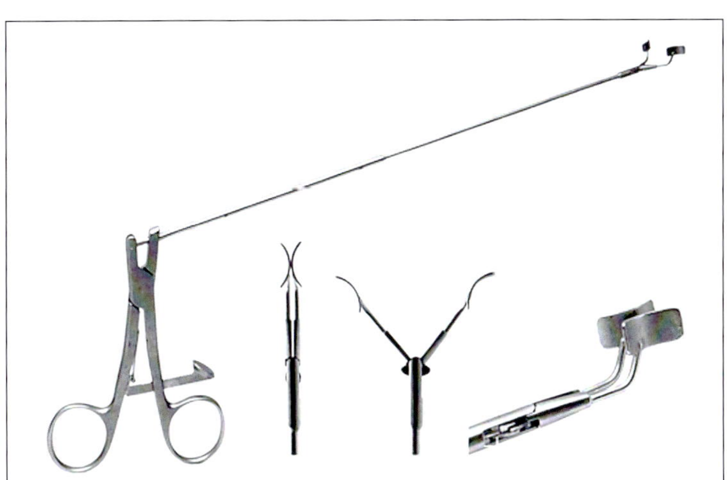

Fig. 2. Vocal fold retractors (inset demonstrates the tip of the instrument).

– Infant, child and adult Lindholm laryngoscopes (Karl Storz) with Benjamin suspension and chest support (Karl Storz)
• Need for a shoulder blade depends on patient age (see figure 1 of the Endoscopic Posterior Cricoid Split with Rib Grafting chapter)

Procedure

• After general mask induction using sevoflurane and gaining intravenous access, the operating room table is turned 90° towards the endoscopist
• If the patient has erupted dentition, a tooth guard is utilized on the anterior maxillary teeth

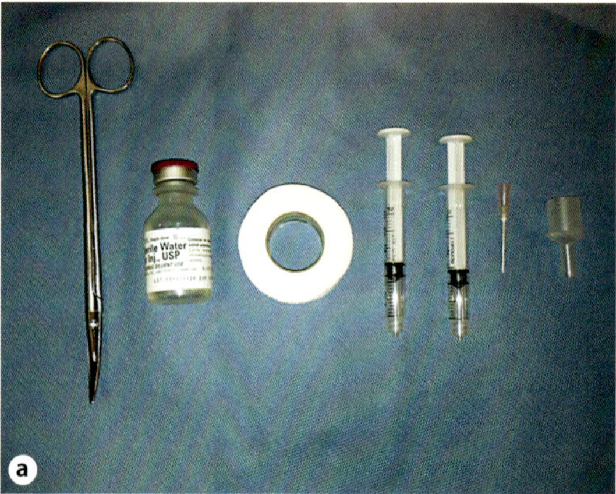 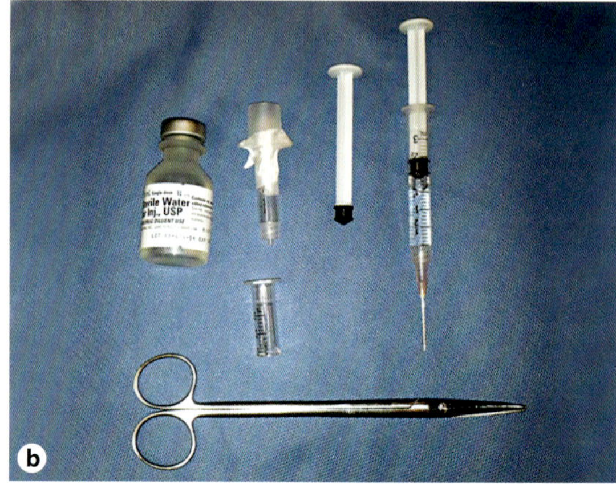

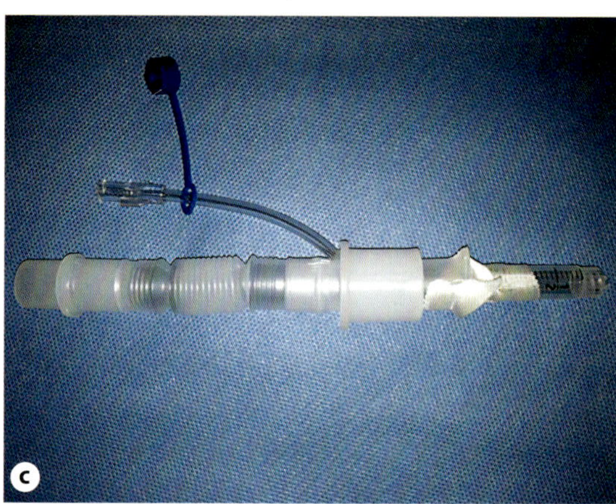

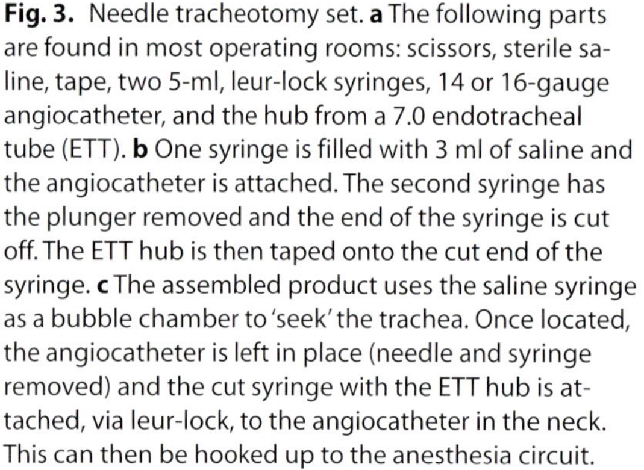

Fig. 3. Needle tracheotomy set. **a** The following parts are found in most operating rooms: scissors, sterile saline, tape, two 5-ml, leur-lock syringes, 14 or 16-gauge angiocatheter, and the hub from a 7.0 endotracheal tube (ETT). **b** One syringe is filled with 3 ml of saline and the angiocatheter is attached. The second syringe has the plunger removed and the end of the syringe is cut off. The ETT hub is then taped onto the cut end of the syringe. **c** The assembled product uses the saline syringe as a bubble chamber to 'seek' the trachea. Once located, the angiocatheter is left in place (needle and syringe removed) and the cut syringe with the ETT hub is attached, via leur-lock, to the angiocatheter in the neck. This can then be hooked up to the anesthesia circuit.

- An appropriate-sized straight blade laryngoscope (either a Miller or Parsons) is placed into the vallecula and the larynx is exposed
- 2 or 4% lidocaine (depending on the child's age and weight) is topically applied with an atomizer to anesthetize the vocal folds and any secretions present are suctioned using a laryngeal microsuction (with thumb suction control)
- The 0° 4 mm × 18 cm Hopkins rod-lens telescope with attached HD camera head is used to evaluate the supraglottis, glottis, subglottis, trachea and primary bronchi (online suppl. video 1)
  - It is the authors' preference to use just the 4-mm telescope if possible in order to achieve the highest resolution image and video. Additionally, it is less bulky when held in the surgeon's hand, and since it is narrower than its associated ventilating bronchoscope, it has the potential for less local tissue irritation and swelling.
  - However, if there is any airway concern for stenosis, or it is an unknown airway with risk of rapid respiratory compromise, a smaller rod-lens telescope may be needed. (0° 2.7 mm × 18 cm, 0° 1.9 mm × 18 cm). Additionally, we have a needle tracheostomy (fig. 3) and tracheotomy set open on the back table prior to starting the procedure as well as a 3.0 or 2.5 endotracheal tube placed over a 1.9-mm Hopkins rod-lens scope (used in a Seldinger fashion) in case there is any airway emergency (fig. 4).

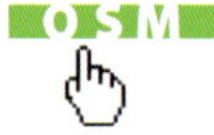

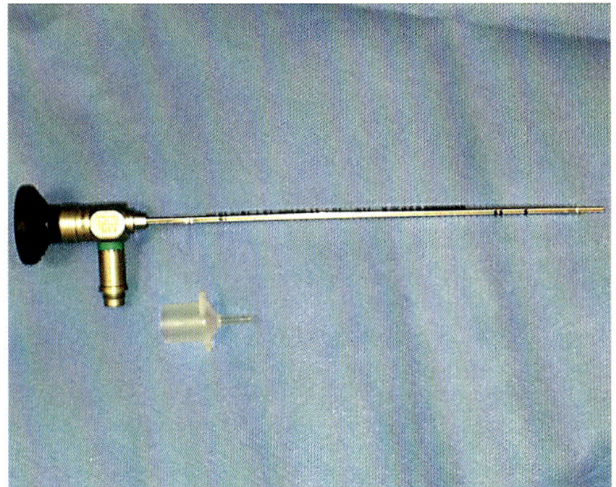

Fig. 4. A 1.9 mm 0° Hopkins rod-lens telescope with 2.5 endotracheal tube placed over it. This can be used to directly visualize placement into the airway via a Seldinger technique.

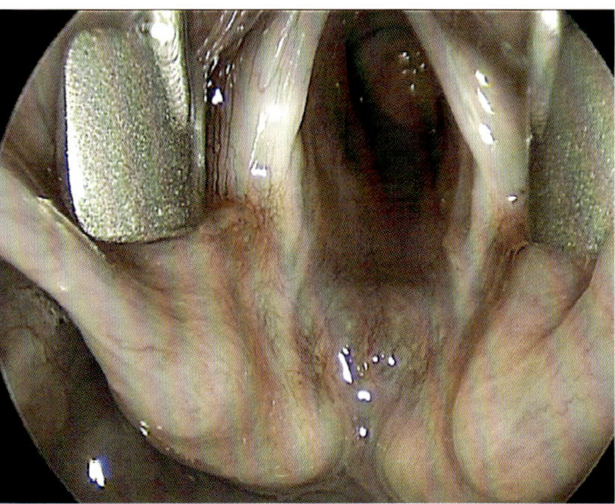

Fig. 6. Type I laryngeal cleft exposed with vocal fold retractors.

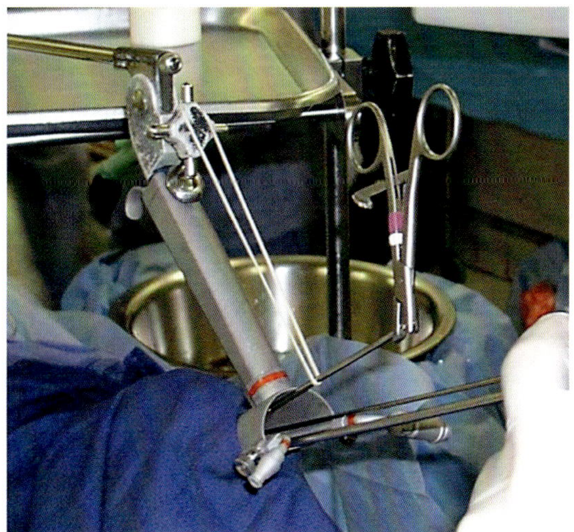

Fig. 5. Suspension laryngoscopy set up with use of vocal fold retractors.

needed, we place the patient into suspension using the Lindholm laryngoscope/Benjamin suspension and chest support (fig. 5)

- The Lindholm vocal cord and false cord retractor is an essential tool for airway evaluation (see the Vocal Fold Retractor video in the Recurrent Respiratory Papillomatosis chapter). It can help with diagnosis and treatment of the following lesions:
  - Laryngeal cleft (fig. 6)
  - Recurrent respiratory papillomatosis (fig. 7)
  - Glottic webs
  - Subglottic stenosis (fig. 8)
  - Proximal tracheal lesions (fig. 9)
  - Airway hemagioma (fig. 10)
  - Pyriform sinus tracts

Postoperative Care

- Depending on other comorbidities (syndromic features, craniofacial dysmorphisms, significant airway stenosis), the patient usually can be discharged the same day as long as he/she is meeting discharge criteria

- If the patient is a neonate or premature with little pulmonary reserve we use an appropriate-size ventilating bronchoscope initially and forgo using just the rod-lens telescope
- If bimanual dexterity for diagnosis or performing a procedure (microlaryngology) is

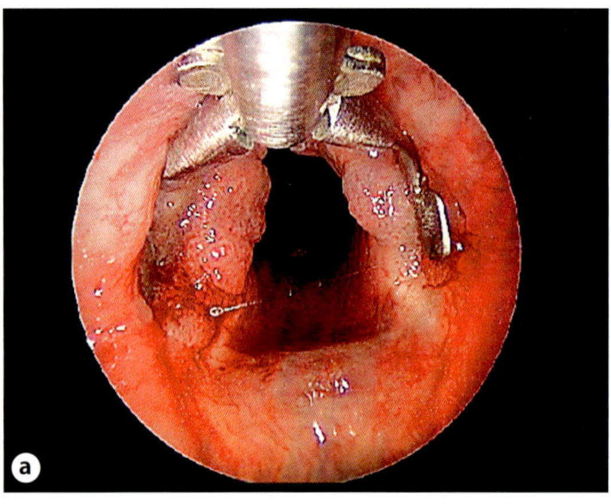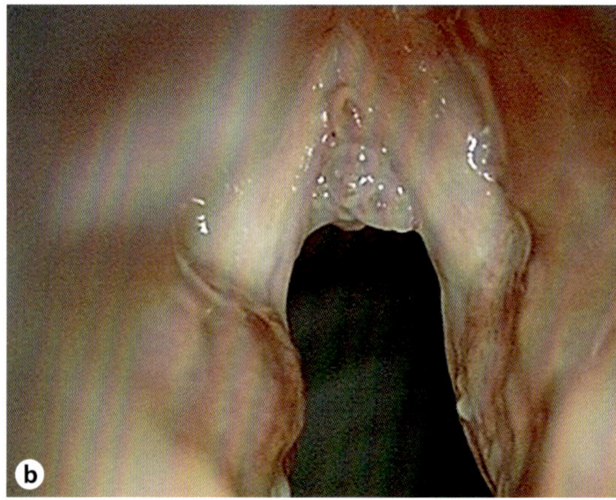

Fig. 7. a Enhanced exposure of RRP on the vocal folds and posterior commissure using vocal fold retractor. **b** Note, flipping the vocal fold retractor 180° will enhance the exposure of the anterior commissure.

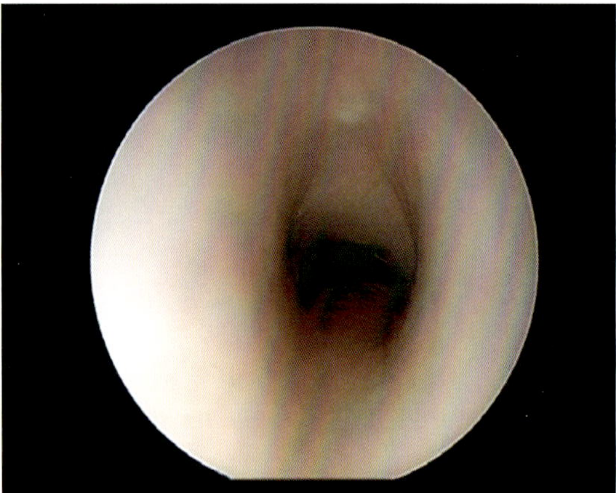

Fig. 8. Subglottic stenosis.

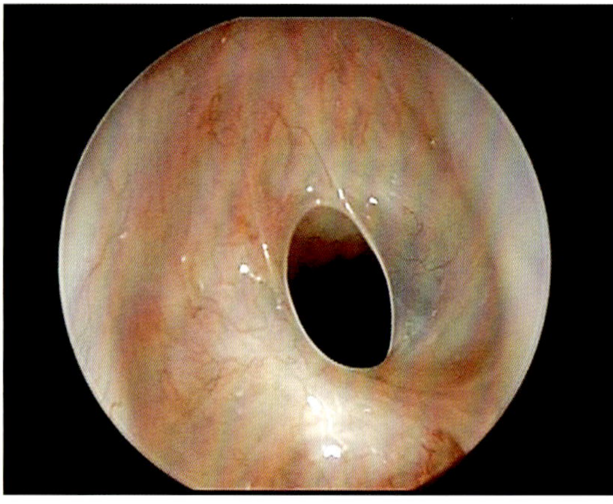

Fig. 9. Proximal tracheal lesion exposed using vocal fold retractor.

– If the patient has significant chronic pulmonary disease, severe asthma, concerns for obstruction after anesthesia, there is a low threshold to observe them overnight
– Patients with a tracheotomy usually can be discharged the same day
• There is minimal pain from this procedure, and most children do well with acetaminophen if any pain medication required

Pearls

• Constant dialogue with your anesthesia provider
• Use of an appropriate-size ventilating bronchoscope if there is poor pulmonary reserve
• If there is any concern for airway stenosis, or it is an unknown airway with risk of rapid respiratory compromise, a smaller rod-lens telescope may be needed. (0° 2.7 mm × 18 cm,

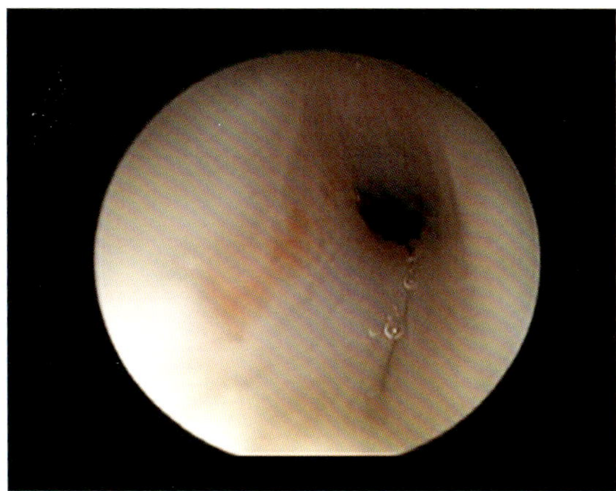

Fig. 10. Airway hemangioma.

0° 1.9 mm × 18 cm). If the smaller scopes do not pass easily, it is unwise to attempt to force through the stenosis as this may turn a stable airway into an unstable one due to resulting edema.

• Having several airway adjuncts ready in case of airway compromise
– The laryngeal mask airway can be very helpful in a situation of difficult ventilation
– Placing a 3.0 or 2.5 endotracheal tube over a 0° 1.9 mm × 18 cm Hopkins rod-lens telescope can be a helpful way to establish a secure airway under direct vision using a Seldinger technique in an emergent airway situation
– Making a needle tracheotomy set and having it ready in case of airway emergency
– A tracheotomy set open on the back table if the surgeon feels an emergent surgical airway might need to be established

References

1 Berci G, Forde KA: History of endoscopy: what lessons have we learned from the past? Surg Endosc 2000;14:5–15.

2 Holinger LD: Diagnostic endoscopy of the pediatric airway. Laryngoscope 1989;99:346–348.

Christopher J. Hartnick, MD
Professor, Department of Otology and Laryngology
Chief, Division of Pediatric Otolaryngology
Director, Pediatric Airway, Voice and Swallowing Center
Chief Quality Officer
Massachusetts Eye and Ear Infirmary, Harvard Medical School
243 Charles Street
Boston, MA 02116 (USA)
E-Mail christopher_hartnick@meei.harvard.edu

Hartnick CJ, Hansen MC, Gallagher TQ (eds): Pediatric Airway Surgery. Adv Otorhinolaryngol. Basel, Karger, 2012, vol 73, pp 26–30

Pediatric Tracheotomy

Thomas Q. Gallagher[a] · Christopher J. Hartnick[b]

[a]LCDR, MC, USN, Department of Otolaryngology, Naval Medical Center Portsmouth, Portsmouth, Va., [b]Department of Otology and Laryngology, Massachusetts Eye & Ear Infirmary, Boston, Mass., USA

Abstract

The procedure of tracheotomy dates back to ancient times. Its use has been adapted in the neonatal and pediatric population over the past half-century. Despite being a life-saving measure, tracheotomy-related mortality rates range from 0.5 to 3.6%, and this procedure is not without significant and sometimes frequent complications. Techniques regarding pediatric tracheotomy vary from surgeon to surgeon and include orientation of skin incision, removal of subcutaneous tissue, orientation of tracheotomy, maturation and stay sutures, as well postoperative care and surveillance. In this chapter, the authors detail their technique for tracheotomy. Surgical pearls for success are highlighted.

The concept of tracheotomy dates back to the days of ancient Greece. Modern-era tracheotomy began with French physician Armand Trousseau in the mid-1800s treating patients with diphtheria-associated dyspnea [1]. Since that time, techniques and indications have evolved with the vast improvements occurring in pediatric and neonatal intensive care medicine.

Despite being a life-saving measure, tracheotomy-related mortality rates range from 0.5 to 3.6%, and this procedure is not without significant and sometimes frequent complications [2–4]. These can include anything from the catastrophic plugging or decannulation to the benign such as suprastomal granuloma and nuisance bleeding. For this reason, infants and children remain intubated longer than adults in order to avoid these potential issues.

Techniques regarding pediatric tracheotomy vary from surgeon to surgeon and include orientation of skin incision, removal of subcutaneous tissue, orientation of tracheotomy, maturation and stay sutures, as well postoperative care and surveillance. A recent practice pattern survey of 225 members (75% return rate) of the American Society of Pediatric Otolaryngology found the following predominating trends in pediatric tracheotomy technique: vertical skin incision, routine removal of subcutaneous fat, maturation of the stoma and routine use of stay sutures and tracheostomy tube ties to secure the tracheostomy tube in place [5].

Relevant Anatomy

- The sternal notch, cricoid cartilage and hyoid bone should be identified and marked with a pen prior to starting the procedure

- As discussed in the anatomy chapter, it is important to note the relationship of the hyoid bone and thyroid cartilage in neonates and infants
  - In this age group, the thyroid cartilage 'telescopes' beneath the hyoid bone (see figure 2 of the Laryngeal Development and Anatomy chapter).
  - This relationship is important because the surgeon cannot rely on palpation of the thyroid notch (i.e. adults) as much as the hyoid bone as a relevant anatomic landmark in pediatric neck surgery

Indications

There are multiple indications for tracheotomy in the pediatric age group with the two most common being chronic ventilation (53%) and airway obstruction (38%) [3].

Contraindications

None.

Anesthesia Considerations

- Communication with the anesthesiologist is crucial during this procedure. As seen often in pediatric aerodigestive surgery, exchanging ventilation tubes from one site to another requires careful collaboration between the surgeon and the anesthesiologist, and a discussion of the steps or flow of the case should be done prior to starting the procedure.
- The oxygen concentration should be reduced as much as possible in an effort to decrease the risk of airway fire during the dissection with electrocautery

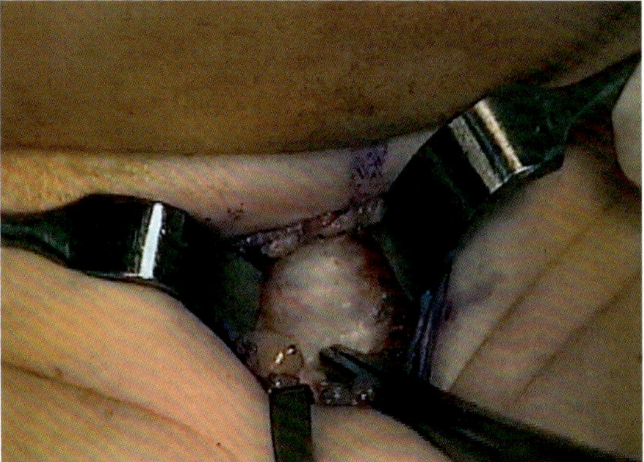

Fig. 1. Retraction both laterally and pushing down into the wound assists the surgeon in preventing erroneous dissection laterally.

Preparation

- Pediatric tracheotomy should be done over a definitive airway under general anesthesia if at all possible
- Several different size tracheotomy tubes should be available
- A shoulder roll is utilized in order to expose the necessary surgical landmarks
- The surgeon should wear a headlight, and loupe magnification can be helpful

Procedure

- A 1- to 2-cm vertical incision is marked out in the midline neck about just inferior to the cricoid
  - Vertical incision is preferred over horizontal due to the ability to extend the incision easily intraoperatively and the lack of redundant skin above and below the tracheostoma allowing recannulation easier
- The wound edges then have the subcutaneous fat removed using electrocautery
- Exposure using small retractors such as a Senn rake or pediatric Ragnell is necessary to keep

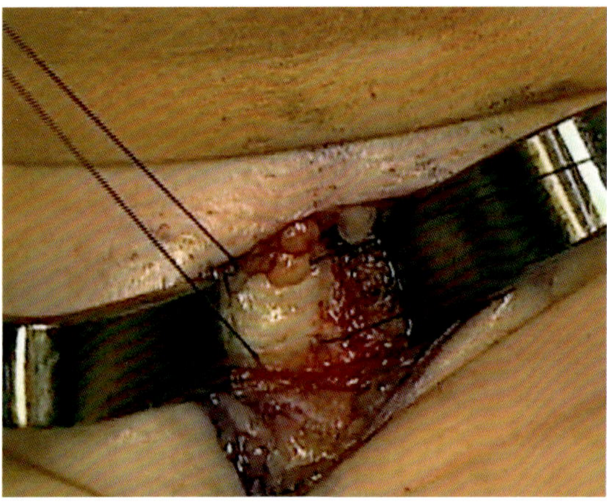

Fig. 2. Stay sutures are placed around the second tracheal ring to help elevate the trachea out of the wound. They will stay in place until the first tracheostomy tube change.

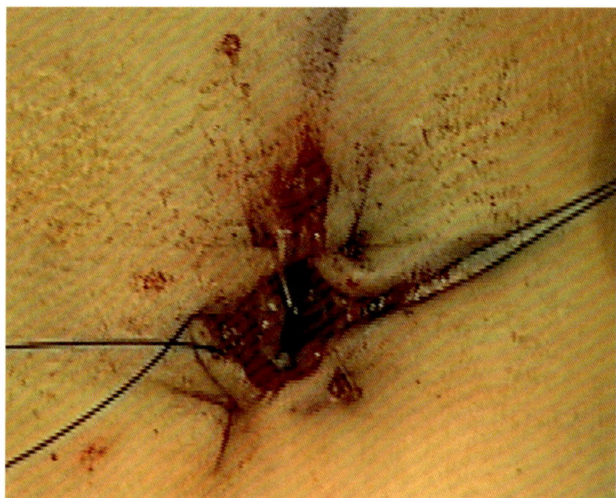

Fig. 3. A view of the matured stoma; note the skin edges are tacked down on to the trachea with little subcutaneous fat in between. This helps to eliminate any potential space and possible 'false passage' in case of accidental decannulation and premature tracheostomy tube change.

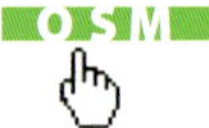

the trachea in constant view during the dissection (fig. 1; online suppl. video 1)

- The strap muscles are divided using electrocautery and the thyroid, if located in the surgical field, is divided with the electrocautery
- Division of the thyroid prevents it from obstructing the trachea in the event of accidental decannulation
- Using bipolar and peanut sponges, the trachea is brought into view and the cricoid is identified
- 4-0 monofilament, non-absorbable suture is placed paramedian at the level of the second and third tracheal rings and secured with mosquito clamps to act as stay sutures (fig. 2)
- This suture should span the cartilaginous tracheal ring
- These are helpful in elevating the trachea out of the wound for the remainder of the case
- These remain in place until the first tracheostomy tube change on postoperative day 5
- After communication with anesthesia, a vertical tracheotomy is made through the second and third tracheal ring

- If the second and third ring cannot be positively identified, it is better to make the tracheotomy lower than higher in order to avoid inadvertent damage to the subglottis
- 4-0 monofilament absorbable suture is then used to 'mature' the tracheostoma. This stitch is thrown in a vertical half-mattress fashion with two superiorly and two inferiorly (fig. 3).
- This will make recannulation easier and prevent the creation of a 'false passage' in the event of accidental decannulation during the first week after tracheotomy
- Use of maturation sutures does not increase the incidence of tracheocutaneous fistulas or granulation tissue formation [6]
- The endotracheal tube is then withdrawn by the anesthesiologist and the tracheostomy tube is placed
- The circuit is switched over and the patient is examined for good chest rise and breath sounds
- The tracheostomy ties are secured around the neck
- The stay sutures are knotted and taped to the chest and marked 'left' and 'right' in case of accidental decannulation

- The shoulder roll is removed and a flexible fiber-optic tracheoscopy is performed to ensure there is adequate distance from the tip of the tracheostomy tube to the carina

Postoperative Care

- Postoperative stay in the intensive care unit until the first tracheostomy tube change
- Humidified trach-collar is an imperative due to the fact that pediatric tracheostomy tubes do not have an inner cannula and can form obstructive crusts very easily
- The first tracheostomy tube change should be performed by the otolaryngology service. This can be performed at the bedside.
- Subsequent tracheostomy tube changes are recommended every 2 weeks
- Depending on the degree of pre-existing airway obstruction, the following airway adjuncts and equipment should be available at the time of the tracheostomy tube change. Otherwise, the surgeon may opt to change the tube in the operating room.
  - Flexible fiber-optic scope
  - Airway cart with different-sized laryngeal mask airways and endotracheal tubes
  - Head light
  - Tracheotomy tube one size smaller than the current tube
  - Cricoid hook and tracheostomy spreader
- Postoperative tracheostomy tube training for parents and caregivers
  - Must change the tracheostomy tube with the nurses at least three times each
  - Must watch an infant CPR video
- There are no current practice guidelines for interval direct laryngoscopy/bronchoscopy for children with tracheostomy tubes. The author's practice pattern is to routinely look in the operating room every 6 months to survey the airway for significant changes (i.e. suprastomal granuloma).

  - The rate of suprastomal granuloma has been reported to be as high as 72–80% [7, 8]
- We recommend immediate endoscopic evaluation of pediatric tracheotomies if any of the following symptoms occur:
  - Severe bleeding from the tracheostomy site
  - Lack of phonation
  - Difficult tracheostomy tube change

Pearls

- Palpation through the wound is done consistently throughout the case in order to maintain anatomical orientation. Due to the relatively small anatomy, it is quite easy to get 'off track' and palpation of the cricoid and trachea will help avoid this error.
  - The authors will remove nasogastric and orogastric feeding tubes prior to performing a tracheotomy to decrease the chance of mistaking the esophagus for the trachea during palpation
- Lateral retraction by the assistant is crucial. It is important that they help bring the airway into view with replacement and advancement of the retractors deep into the wound bed.
- Placement of stay sutures serve two purposes:
  - During the procedure, they elevate the trachea out of the wound prior to entering the airway. It is imperative to avoid subglottic injury by incorrect placement of the tracheostomy tube. Placement of these stay sutures gives the airway surgeon better control of the airway in order to correctly identify the surgical landmarks necessary to place the tracheostomy tube correctly.
  - When left in place, taped to the chest, they serve to assist in replacing the tracheostomy tube if accidental decannulation occurs in the immediate postoperative period
- Post-tracheotomy direct laryngoscopy and bronchoscopy are important to confirm good placement of the tracheostomy tube.

References

1 Peumery JJ: Armand Trousseau (1801–1867), French physician par excellence. Hist Sci Med 2003;2:151–156.
2 Wetmore FR, Handler SD, Postic WP: Pediatric tracheostomy – experience during the past decade. Ann Otol Rhinol Laryngol 1982;91:628–633.
3 Wetmore RF, Marsh RR, Thompson ME, et al: Pediatric tracheotomy: changing a procedure? Ann Otol Rhinol Laryngol 1999;108:695–699.
4 Carr MM, Poje CP, Kingston L, et al: Complications in pediatric tracheostomies. Laryngoscope 2001;111:1925–1928.
5 Ruggiero FP, Carr MM: Infant tracheotomy, results of a survey regarding technique. Arch Otolaryngol Head Neck Surg 2008;134:263–267.
6 Park JY, Suskind DL, Munz HR, Lusk RP: Maturation of the pediatric tracheostomy stoma: effect on complications. Ann Otol Rhinol Laryngol 1999;108:1115–1119.
7 Rosenfeld RM, Stool SE: Should granulomas be excised in children with long-term tracheotomy? Arch Otolaryngol Head Neck Surg 1992;118:1323–1327.
8 Benjamin B, Curley JW: Infant tracheotomy – endoscopy and decannulation. Int J Pediatr Otolaryngol 1990;20:113–121.

Christopher J. Hartnick, MD
Professor, Department of Otology and Laryngology
Chief, Division of Pediatric Otolaryngology
Director, Pediatric Airway, Voice and Swallowing Center
Chief Quality Officer
Massachusetts Eye and Ear Infirmary, Harvard Medical School
243 Charles Street
Boston, MA 02116 (USA)
E-Mail christopher_hartnick@meei.harvard.edu

Hartnick CJ, Hansen MC, Gallagher TQ (eds): Pediatric Airway Surgery. Adv Otorhinolaryngol. Basel, Karger, 2012, vol 73, pp 31–38

Laryngotracheal Reconstruction

Thomas Q. Gallagher[a] · Christopher J. Hartnick[b]

[a]LCDR, MC, USN, Department of Otolaryngology, Naval Medical Center Portsmouth, Portsmouth, Va., [b]Department of Otology and Laryngology, Massachusetts Eye & Ear Infirmary, Boston, Mass., USA

Abstract

Laryngotracheal reconstruction (LTR) along with cricotracheal resection and thyrotracheal anastomosis has become the standard of care for symptomatic subglottic stenosis in the pediatric age group. Success rates in achieving decannulation or avoiding tracheotomy approach 90%. Fearon and Cotton introduced pediatric LTR in 1972 using cartilage interposition grafting. The procedure has evolved to include a variety of techniques for expanding the laryngotracheal complex to obtain a stable airway of sufficient size for respiration. In this chapter, the authors will describe their single and double-stage technique for LTR highlighting surgical pearls necessary for success.

The surgical treatment of subglottic stenosis (SGS) using cartilage interposition grafting was pioneered by Fearon and Cotton in 1972 [1]. This landmark airway expansion technique, which we will refer to as pediatric laryngotracheal reconstruction (LTR), was created in response to a rise in cases of

neonatal acquired SGS. In 1965, McDonald and Stocks [2] published their technique for long-term intubation for reversible pulmonary disease in neonates. Although the advent of this technique was a paradigm shift for survival in neonates, the presence of an endotracheal tube (ETT) in the subglottis for long periods of time increases the risk for circumferential scaring at the narrowest segment of the airway in infants, the cricoid.

In addition to an acquired type, SGS can occur in congenital forms as well. Congenital SGS represents a continuum of incomplete or altered embryologic recanalization of the primitive laryngopharynx. This can range from complete failure of recanalization to a mild shape disturbance (elliptical shape with prominent posterior shelves). This type is more rare and usually less severe than the acquired type.

Regardless of etiology, initial management of SGS can vary from observation to bypassing the stenosis distally with a tracheostomy tube depending on the patient's symptoms. Children with tracheotomies who fail to decannulate are candidates for LTR. Decannulation rates for this procedure approach 90% [3]. In this chapter, the authors will discuss both single- and double-stage LTR with emphasis on preoperative preparation/evaluation, surgical technique and surgical pearls for success.

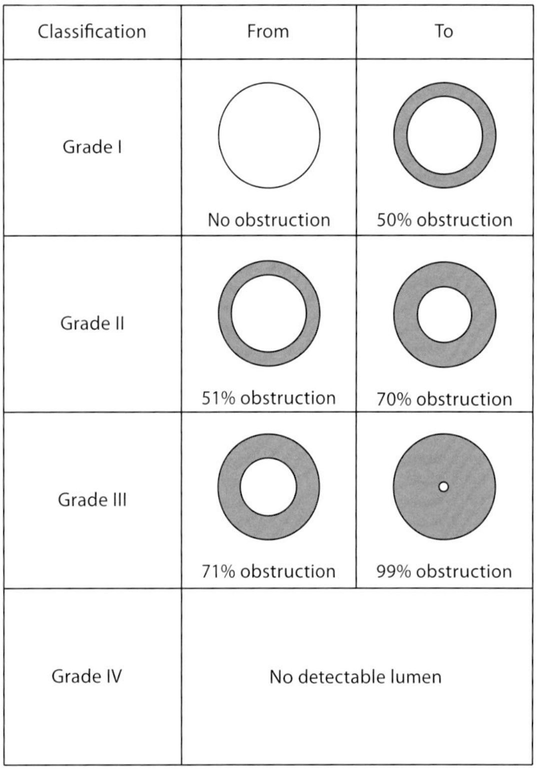

Classification	From	To
Grade I	No obstruction	50% obstruction
Grade II	51% obstruction	70% obstruction
Grade III	71% obstruction	99% obstruction
Grade IV	No detectable lumen	

Fig.1. Myer-Cotton Classification System for SGS (Reprinted with kind permission from [4]).

Relevant Anatomy

For relevant anatomy, see the Laryngeal Development and Anatomy chapter (pp 1–11).

Indications

- Moderate to severe SGS (acquired or congenital). Not based solely on Myer-Cotton staging but rather symptomatology as well.
- Myer-Cotton Classification System for SGS (fig. 1) [4]:
  - Grade I – no obstruction to 50% obstruction
  - Grade II – 50% obstruction to 70% obstruction
  - Grade III – 71% obstruction to 99% obstruction
  - Grade IV – no detectable lumen

- Particularly indicated (as opposed to CTR) when there is:
- Glottic and subglottic stenosis
- SGS that is too close to the vocal folds to allow for a safe superior plane of dissection to be developed

Contraindications

- Severe tracheomalacia
- Uncontrolled gastroesophageal reflux or reactive airway disease
- Active eosinophilic esophagitis
- Tracheostomy tube dependence due to chronic pulmonary disease or neurologic impairment including oxygen dependence

Anesthesia Considerations

- Communication is paramount throughout the procedure due to the fact that the ETT changes positions and is removed several times during the case
- A sterile anesthesia circuit is necessary for a portion of the procedure

Preparation

- Direct laryngoscopy and rigid bronchoscopy to evaluate severity of SGS and to size the airway
- Airway sizing is done with an uncuffed ETT
- The age-appropriate ETT is determined by using the following formula: (age + 16)/4. A leak test to 20 cm H_2O pressure is used to determine accurate size. For example, a 4-year-old child's airway should safely accommodate a 5.0 ETT.
- Effective neck extension with a shoulder roll is necessary
- If the surgeon is confident that an LTR will be the procedure performed, then costal cartilage

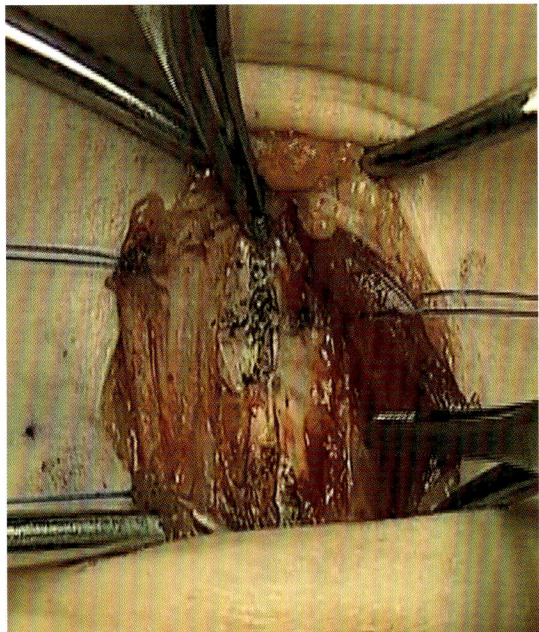

Fig. 2. Forceps placed in thyroid notch for orientation. Laryngofissure is scored in a cruciform pattern with electrocautery.

harvest is done prior to the open airway procedure to limit the risk of wound infection. If there is a question of whether costal cartilage grafting will be required or whether the procedure will be an LTR or CTR, then the rib harvest is planned after the airway is opened. The cartilage is carved and placed in sterile saline solution until needed (see associated chapter on cartilage harvest).

Procedure

- Transverse cervical skin incision over the cricoid (online suppl. video 1). Center around the tracheostomy stoma if planning single-stage surgery
- Elevate skin flaps in the subcutaneous plane superiorly to the thyroid notch and inferiorly to the level of obstruction
- Gelpi retractors are placed
- Divide strap muscles and retract using 4-0 nonabsorbable monofilament sutures. Skeletonize the thyroid cartilage and upper trachea
- Place 4-0 nonabsorbable monofilament sutures into the trachea inferior to the tracheotomy to gain positive control of the distal airway
- Place 4-0 non-absorbable monofilament sutures on either side of the proposed vertical cricoid split
- If a laryngofissure is planned, use the electro-cautery to mark vertical midline on the thyroid cartilage as well as a horizontal hash mark to allow for precise reapproximation upon completion of surgery (fig. 2)
- A 6900 Beaver blade is utilized for the anterior cricoid split. A Jake hemostat is then placed through the incision to distract the cricoid split. The incision is then carried superiorly to the thyroid cartilage and inferior to the first tracheal ring. If the stenosis is involving the first tracheal ring, then it is divided as well.
- Laryngofissure
- Performed using the 6900 beaver blade, divide the anterior perichondrium and thyroid cartilage but not the posterior perichondrium
- Using a Jake hemostat, the true vocal folds are identified. At this point, the anterior commissure is divided sharply.
- Endoscopic assistance with an assistant operating a 0° telescope can be utilized in order to directly visualize the division of the anterior commissure. This is helpful if there is a grade 4 stenosis or for revision cases.
- The area of stenosis is then assessed (fig. 3)
- A tuberculin syringe with a 27-gauge needle is then used to infiltrate the posterior tracheal mucosa with 1% lidocaine with 1:100,000 epinephrine. Less than 0.5 ml is usually needed.
- The posterior cricoid split is performed using a right-angled hemostat to apply adequate counter-traction (in a posterior-lateral fashion).

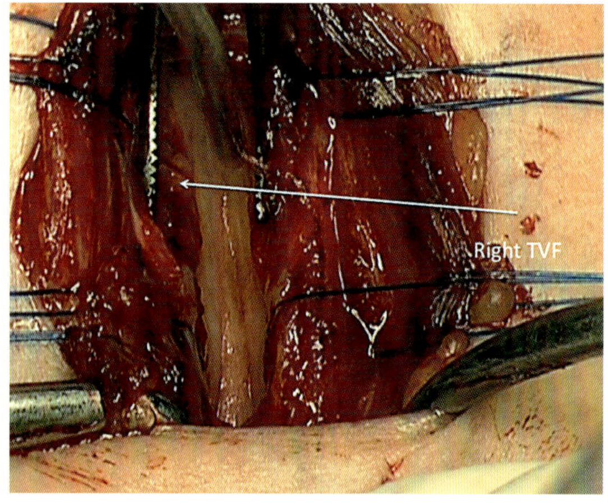

Fig. 3. Following laryngofissure, the anatomy is exposed and the subglottis is evaluated.

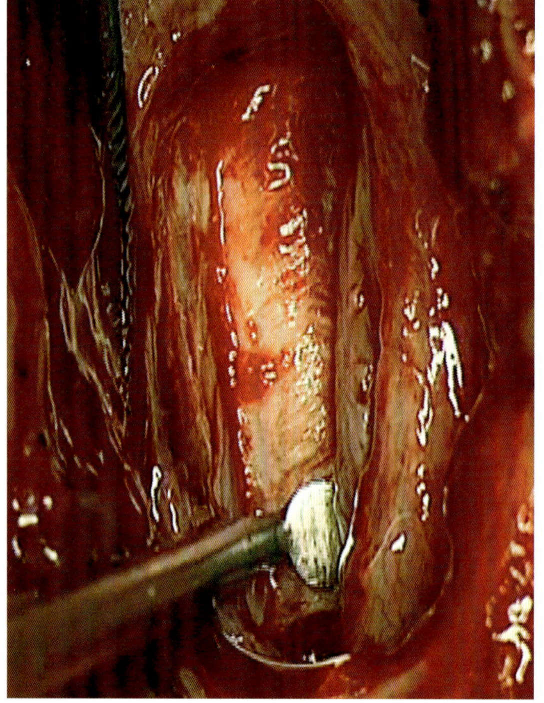

Fig. 4. An otologic round knife is used to undermine the posterior surface of the cricoid cartilage after the posterior cricoid split is performed. The raphe and oblique fibers of the posterior cricoarytenoid muscle can be seen deep to the round knife.

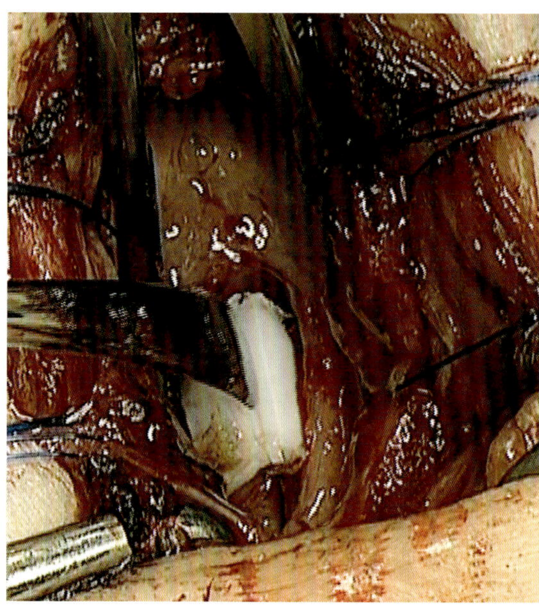

Fig. 5. A broad-based instrument is used to advance the posterior graft into position.

The 6900 Beaver blade is then used to divide the complete posterior cricoid until a release is appreciated and the muscle fibers below can be seen. An assistant providing suction with a 5 Frazier-tipped suction is essential to maintain good visualization.

- A medium sized otologic round knife is then used to undermine the posterior surface of the cricoid along the posterior cricoid split in order to accommodate the posterior cartilage graft (fig. 4)
- The posterior cartilage graft is placed. A broad-based instrument (i.e. Freer elevator) is helpful in applying pressure to 'snap' the graft in place (fig. 5, 6).
- The laryngofissure (if performed) is closed prior to airway sizing and anterior graft placement. This is done utilizing 4-0 absorbable monofilament suture. The horizontal hash marks are lined up and a vertical mattress suture is thrown (far-far, near-near) in a submucosal fashion (fig. 7). The remainder of the thyroid

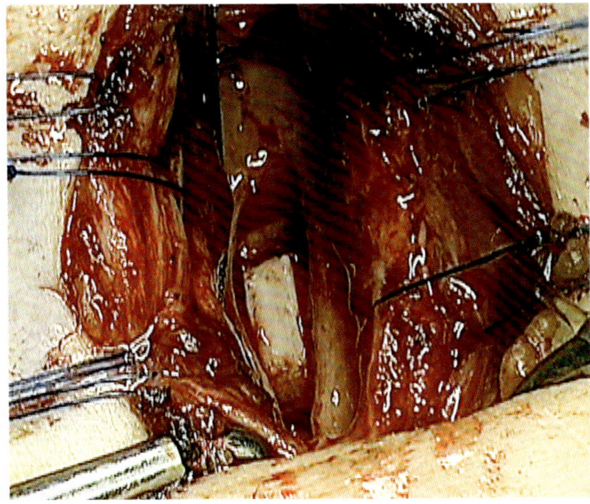

Fig. 6. Posterior graft in position.

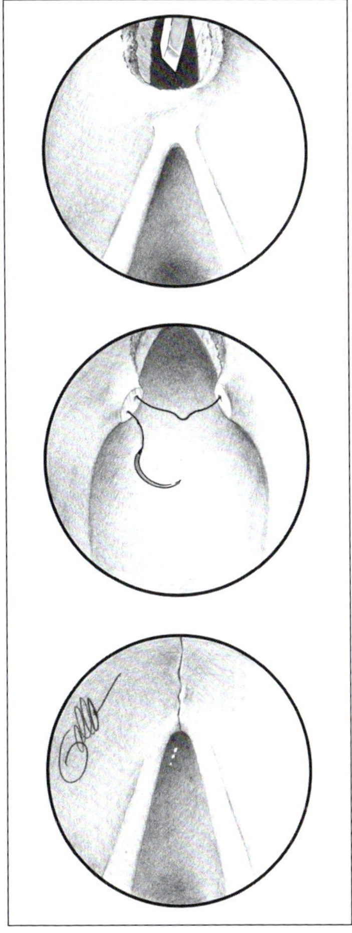

Fig. 7. The reapproximation of the anterior commissure is demonstrated.

cartilage is reapproximated with simple interrupted 4-0 braided absorbable sutures.

- The airway is then sized to an age-appropriate ETT, and the patient has a nasotracheal tube placed
- An appropriate-sized anterior graft is then placed (fig. 8). It is sutured into position with 4-0 braided absorbable sutures (4 or 6 depending on size of the graft) thrown in a horizontal mattress fashion.
- All sutures are thrown and carefully orientated on a blue towel prior to tying down in order to avoid crossing suture lines
- The wound is closed in a layered fashion. Fibrin glue sealant is placed over the trachea prior to closure of the strap muscles. A rubber band drain is utilized for prevention of subcutaneous emphysema and hematoma/seroma formation.
- Double-staged procedure:
- Transverse cervical skin incision is modified. It is placed superior to the tracheostomy tube over the cricoid cartilage.
- After placing the posterior costal cartilage graft, an appropriate sized stent is placed and secured into position. Choice of the ideal stent material varies, and is beyond the scope of

this chapter; however, the authors favor the following:

- A cut Montgomery T-tube with the superior end sutured closed
- An Aboulker stent
- If the airway is large enough (age >5 years old) and there is concern for glottis stenosis, a Montgomery T-tube may be used
- Using the formula for age-appropriate pediatric ETT (see above) and extrapolating the outer diameter of the ETT, an appropriate-sized stent is chosen

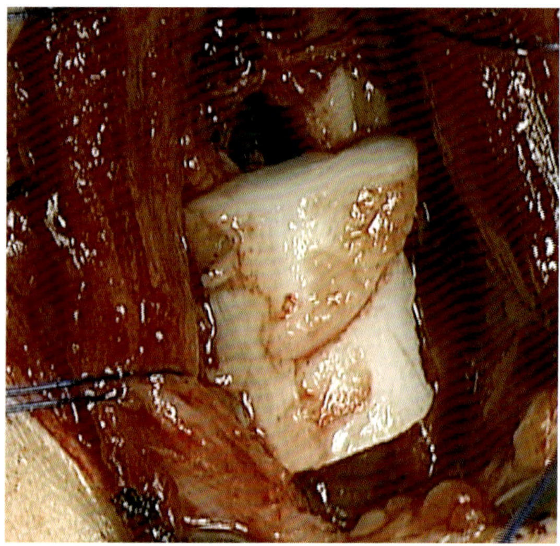

Fig. 8. Anterior graft positioned into anterior cricoid split.

- The stent should be placed so it is above the level of the true vocal folds but not too 'high' to cause aspiration. The inferior portion of the stent should be abutting the tracheostomy tube. Any cut edges of the stent should be made soft and smooth.
- The shoulder roll should be removed when measuring and placing the stent
- The stent is secured using a 2-0 nonabsorbable monofilament suture passed though the following structures: strap muscles, trachea, stent, contralateral tracheal wall, and contralateral strap muscles. It is secured at the time of closing over an 18-gauge angio-catheter left in the subcutaneous tissues.
- By convention, the knot for the stent suture is placed to the patient's right in order to facilitate its location at the time of stent removal

Postoperative Care

- Single stage <3–4 years old:
- Nasogastric feeding tube is utilized

- Nasotracheal intubation for 3 days to 1 week (depending upon whether it is an anterior graft, posterior graft, or anteroposterior grafts) in the PICU with paralysis and sedation incorporating medication holidays as tolerated
- Prophylactic reflux medication for 3 months
- Wean sedation medications 24 h prior to extubation in the OR. The use of dexmedetomidine may be helpful in this process.
- Intravenous steroids initiated 24 h prior to extubation and continued 24 h after extubation
- A swallow evaluation is performed to determine diet. Patients who had a laryngofissure undergo modified barium swallow. All others may undergo bedside evaluation.
- A second direct laryngoscopy and bronchoscopy is performed at the 2-week mark prior to hospital discharge. At this time, balloon dilation may be utilized.
- Single stage >3–4 years old:
- Paralysis may not be necessary in this age group due to their ability to manage breathing through a nasotracheal tube while awake
- The remainder of the care is similar to the above
- Double stage:
- The patient is awoken at the end of the case and transferred to the PICU for overnight observation
- Pain control and supportive care
- A modified barium swallow is performed prior to initiating diet in order to ascertain aspiration risk
- The stent is removed in the OR at the one-week period, and follow-up laryngoscopies are performed similar to the single stage patients

Pearls

- Until one identifies the thyroid notch, one cannot be completely sure of their location along the laryngotracheal skeleton. This especially holds true in revision surgery.

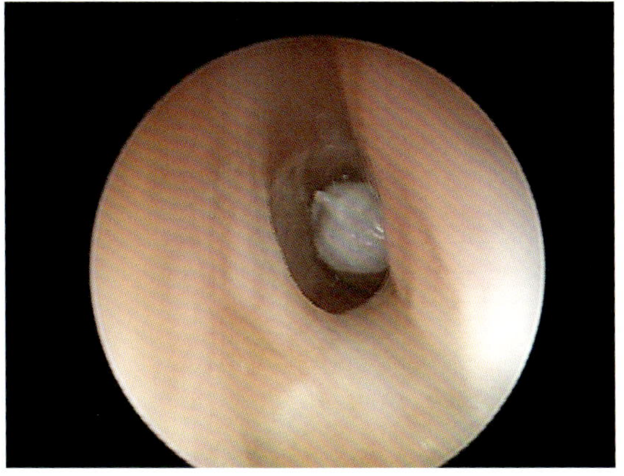

Fig. 9. Preoperative direct laryngoscopy demonstrating grade III SGS and a suprastomal granuloma distally.

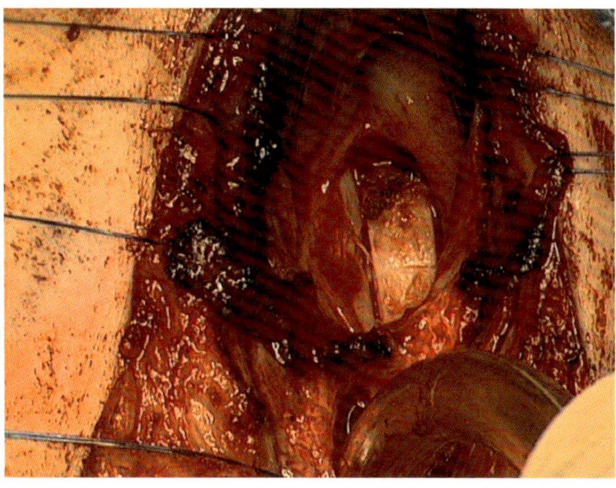

Fig. 11. Intraoperative photo showing the posterior graft in place.

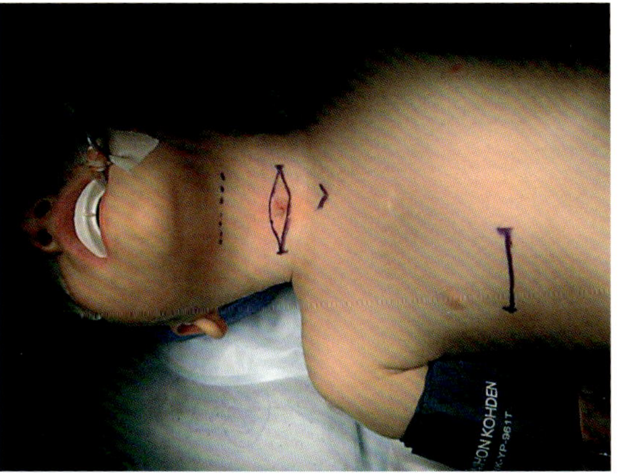

Fig. 10. Preoperative marking and positioning is demonstrated. The dotted line represents the location of the hyoid bone.

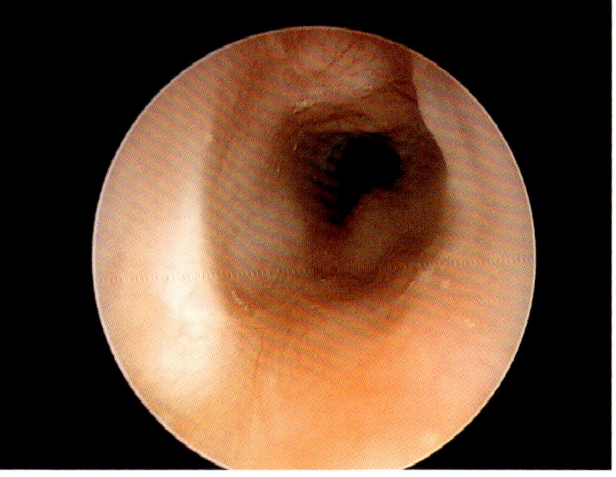

Fig. 12. Two months after operation, the graft site is well mucosalized. Distally, some tracheomalacia is appreciated.

- Keep 4-0 retraction sutures organized so that any sutures retracting the airway are identifiable. In our OR, we use cut pieces of the magnetic instrument pad to separate muscle retraction sutures from airway retraction sutures.
- Keep in mind the anatomical location of the hyoid bone in the infant. Remember the thyroid cartilage 'telescopes' under the hyoid bone.
- If this is a reconstruction performed on a patient without a tracheotomy (i.e. congenital SGS with cyanosis during upper respiratory symptoms) then a temporary intraoperative tracheostomy is placed below the area of stenosis at about the third tracheal ring using any ETT. It is removed and sutured closed at the end of the case using 4-0 absorbable suture. Do not connect the tracheotomy with the reconstruction site or one might risk destabilizing the trachea leading to tracheomalacia.

- Posterior cricoid split: The counter-traction provided by the right-angled hemostat is essential to a successful split. It should allow the cartilage to fall away as the blade divides it.
- The shoulder roll should be removed prior to measuring and placing a double-staged airway stent

Case Presentation

A 2-year-old male, former 26-week premature infant, presented with acquired SGS. He suffered a left true vocal fold paralysis secondary to PDA ligation during his neonatal hospitalization. He received a tracheotomy for continued respiratory distress 2 months after birth. On direct laryngoscopy and bronchoscopy his airway was noted to have posterior glottic stenosis and was sized as a grade III SGS (fig. 9). Laryngeal electromyography demonstrated no motor unit action potentials on the left true vocal cord. A single-staged LTR was planned with 1-week intubation, sedation and paralysis in the PICU (fig. 10). Intraoperatively, an anterior and posterior cricoid split was performed along with a posterior costal cartilage interposition graft (fig. 11). His hospital course was uneventful, and he was extubated at the 1-week mark and discharged at the 2-week mark after repeat direct laryngoscopy/bronchoscopy. A repeat bronchoscopy at the 4-week postoperative mark as well as the 8-week postoperative mark (fig. 12) demonstrated a well-mucosalized graft and a patent subglottis. There was some short segment tracheomalacia present for which he remained asymptomatic.

References

1 Fearon B, Cotton R: Surgical correction of subglottic stenosis of the larynx. Preliminary report of an experimental surgical technique. Ann Otol Rhinol Laryngol 1972;81:508–513.

2 McDonald IH, Stocks JG: Prolonged nasotracheal intubation. A review of its development in a paediatric hospital. Br J Anaesth 1965;37:161–173.

3 Cotton RT, Gray SD, Miller RP: Update of the Cincinnati experience in pediatric laryngotracheal reconstruction. Laryngoscope 1989;99:1111–1116.

4 Myer CM III, OConnor DM, Cotton RT: Proposed grading system for subglottic stenosis based on endotracheal tube sizes. Ann Otol Rhinol Laryngol 1994;103:319–323.

Christopher J. Hartnick, MD
Professor, Department of Otology and Laryngology
Chief, Division of Pediatric Otolaryngology
Director, Pediatric Airway, Voice and Swallowing Center
Chief Quality Officer
Massachusetts Eye and Ear Infirmary, Harvard Medical School
243 Charles Street
Boston, MA 02116 (USA)
E-Mail christopher_hartnick@meei.harvard.edu

Hartnick CJ, Hansen MC, Gallagher TQ (eds): Pediatric Airway Surgery. Adv Otorhinolaryngol. Basel, Karger, 2012, vol 73, pp 39–41

Costal Cartilage Harvest

Thomas Q. Gallagher[a] · Christopher J. Hartnick[b]

[a]LCDR, MC, USN, Department of Otolaryngology, Naval Medical Center Portsmouth, Portsmouth, Va., [b]Department of Otology and Laryngology, Massachusetts Eye & Ear Infirmary, Boston, Mass., USA

Abstract

Cartilage interposition grafting for treatment of subglottic stenosis was pioneered by Fearon and Cotton in 1972. Costal cartilage is the preferred source for graft material in most cases. In this section, the authors highlight the surgical technique for cartilage graft harvest with discussion of surgical pearls necessary for success.

Relevant Anatomy

- Structures divided during dissection (superficial to deep):
- Skin and subcutaneous fat
- Muscle fibers of the pectoralis major muscle, rectus abdominus muscle and external oblique muscle
- Depending on which rib harvested and age/muscle development of patient
- Perichondrium of cartilaginous rib

Indications

Subglottis stenosis requiring cartilage augmentation.

Contraindications

- Age less than 1 year – rib cartilage may be too small to carve adequately for an insert graft
- Osteogenesis imperfecta

Anesthesia Considerations

Communication with your anesthesia provider regarding the chance of pneumothorax with this procedure.

Preparation

- A 4-cm incision is marked out of the desired rib. Injection with 1% lidocaine with 1:100,000 epinephrine is utilized.
- Rib selection is based on obtaining the most flat and straight piece of cartilage that can be obtained. This usually is the 5th or 6th rib.
- Gender is important to consider with making incision. Placement of the incision in the

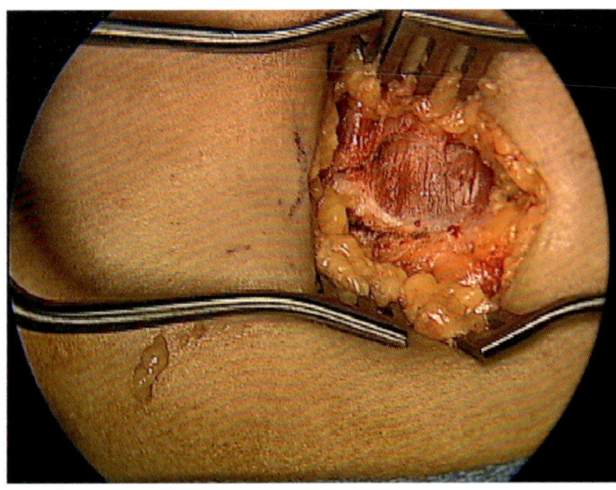

Fig. 1. Muscular layer is exposed.

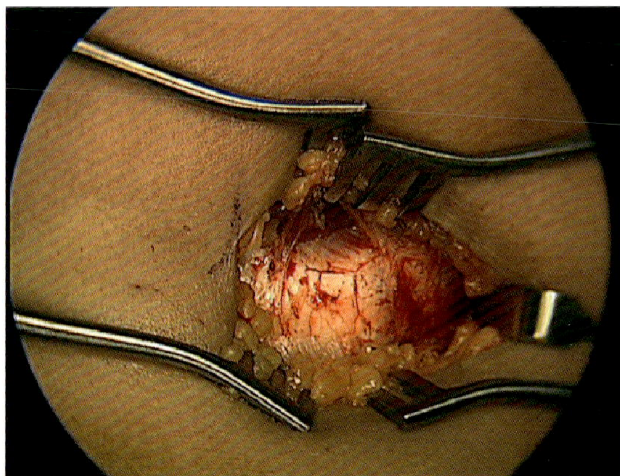

Fig. 2. Perichondrium of rib is exposed.

mammary crease is considered for female patients.

- If the need for autogenous cartilage is known prior to surgery, the harvest is performed prior to opening the airway in order to maintain sterile technique for the chest wound

Procedure

- Sharp dissection through the skin is carried into the subcutaneous fat
- Blunt dissection over the selected rib is performed with a hemostat and electrocautery
- Palpation of the desired rib is done throughout the procedure in order to avoid erroneous dissection
- Muscle fibers are divided with electrocautery (fig. 1; online suppl. video 1)
- The rib is exposed with the use of blunt dissection from peanut sponges (fig. 2). Self-retaining retractors are utilized.
- The rib is examined to ensure sufficient length (>2 cm) and shape. The bony-cartilaginous junctions are identified.

- The inferior and superior edges of the rib are cauterized to help reduce bleeding
- Along the inferior and superior edges, the perichondrium is sharply incised
- Subperichondrial dissection with a Cottle elevator is initiated through these incisions. The dissection is then continued with a Freer elevator. Care is taken to make contact with the undersurface of the rib the entire time.
- Once the inferior and superior subperichondrial dissections are complete, the lateral bony-cartilaginous junction (blue in color) is identified (fig. 3)
- The lateral rib is incised sharply over the Freer
- The remainder of the posterior rib dissection is completed under direct vision. This is accomplished with the surgeon in the seated position.
- The medial incision is made once ensuring at least 2 cm of cartilage is harvested
- Again, this is done over the Freer to avoid injury to the structures below
- Once removed, the rib is placed on the back table in saline solution
- The wound is filled with sterile saline solution, and a Valsalva maneuver to 30 cm water

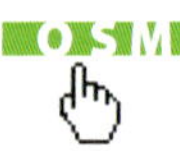

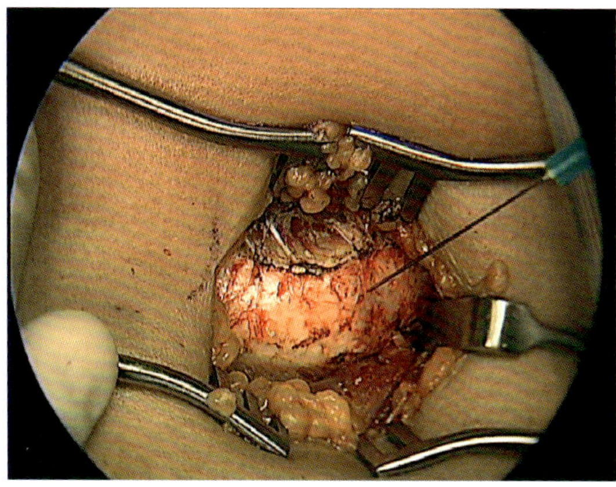

Fig. 3. The rib is exposed and the 'blue line' is identified with the needle. This is the bony-cartilaginous junction.

pressure is performed to ensure the thoracic cavity was not violated

- The wound is checked for hemostasis and closed in a layered fashion over a rubber band drain using absorbable braided suture. Approximation of the muscular layer is necessary.

Postoperative Care

- A portable chest X-ray is obtained in the recovery room or intensive care unit to ensure there is no pneumothorax

- The rubber band drain is usually removed on postoperative day 1 or 2

Pearls

- The patient's gender is kept in mind when marking the incision
- The size and shape of the rib are more important than which rib number
- Use of electrocautery on the inferior and superior edges of the rib prior to sharply incising will help reduce nuisance bleeding
- During subperichondrial dissection with the Freer, contact with the posterior surface of the rib is essential in order to prevent entry into the thoracic cavity
- Identification of the 'blue line' laterally prior to dividing the rib will help to obtain the largest graft possible
- The surgeon in the seated position will facilitate dissection of the posterior perichondrium of the rib

Christopher J. Hartnick, MD
Professor, Department of Otology and Laryngology
Chief, Division of Pediatric Otolaryngology
Director, Pediatric Airway, Voice and Swallowing Center
Chief Quality Officer
Massachusetts Eye and Ear Infirmary, Harvard Medical School
243 Charles Street
Boston, MA 02116 (USA)
E-Mail christopher_hartnick@meei.harvard.edu

Hartnick CJ, Hansen MC, Gallagher TQ (eds): Pediatric Airway Surgery. Adv Otorhinolaryngol. Basel, Karger, 2012, vol 73, pp 42–49

Cricotracheal Resection and Thryotracheal Anastomosis

Thomas Q. Gallagher[a] · Christopher J. Hartnick[b]

[a]LCDR, MC, USN, Department of Otolaryngology, Naval Medical Center Portsmouth, Portsmouth, Va., [b]Department of Otology and Laryngology, Massachusetts Eye & Ear Infirmary, Boston, Mass., USA

Abstract

Cricotracheal resection and thryotracheal anastomosis along with laryngotracheal reconstruction have become the standard of care for symptomatic subglottic stenosis in the pediatric age group with decannulation rates approaching 90%. The procedure is ideal for children with subglottic stenosis several millimeters distal to the true vocal cords and can be extended to include costal interposition grafting if necessary. In this chapter, the authors describe the surgical techniques necessary for successful resection and reanastomosis.

Cricotracheal resection and thryotracheal anastomosis (CTR) along with laryngotracheal reconstruction (LTR) have become the standard of care for symptomatic subglottic stenosis in the pediatric age group [1–4]. Success rates in achieving decannulation or avoiding tracheotomy approach 90% [5]. This technique offers the potential of removing the scarred portion of the

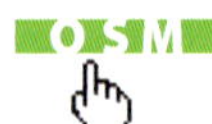

The views expressed in this article are those of the authors and do not necessarily reflect the official policy or position of the Department of the Navy, Department of Defense, or the United States Government.

Thomas Q. Gallagher is a military service member. This work was prepared as part of his official duties. Title 17 .S.C. 105 provides that 'Copyright protection under this title is not available for any work of the United States Government.' Title 17 U.S.C. 101 defines a United States Government work as a work prepared by a military service member or employee of the United States Government as part of that person's official duties.

airway and prevents the need for harvesting a rib graft.

In 1974, Gerwat and Bryce [6] were the first to describe the CTR procedure in a child. Monnier et al. [7, 8] further advanced the procedure in the 1990s, and it has continued to evolve over the past decade.

The CTR is utilized for symptomatic subglottic stenosis that is isolated from the true vocal folds by greater than several millimeters. If the lesion is not purely subglottic, it may be combined with a posterior cricoid split and costal cartilage interposition grafting (extended CTR). CTR has also been utilized for recurrent or persisting subglottic stenosis after previous LTRs. The CTR may be performed in a single-staged or double-staged manner depending on several factors including the child's neurologic and cardiopulmonary status as well as if the procedure is an extended CTR (online suppl. video 1).

CTR is a more technically difficult procedure than LTR. Possible risks include recurrent laryngeal nerve injury (<3%) and anastomotic dehiscence (5%) [7]. Concerns for inhibition of laryngeal growth have been shown to be unfounded in several retrospective papers following CTR patients over a 10-year period [8–10].

Indications

- Moderate to severe subglottic stenosis (acquired or congenital). Not based solely on Cotton-Myer staging but rather symptomatology as well.
- Subglottic stenosis must be distinct from the vocal folds ($\geq$3 mm)
- Recurrent or persistent subglottic stenosis after previous LTR

Contraindications

- Uncontrolled gastroesophageal reflux or reactive airway disease
- Active eosinophilic esophagitis
- Tracheostomy tube dependence due to chronic pulmonary disease, including oxygen dependence, or neurologic impairment
- Subglottic stenosis with glottic involvement

Anesthesia Considerations

- Communication is key due to the fact that the endotracheal tube (ETT) changes positions and is removed several times during the case
- The patient may have a tracheotomy tube, thus changing the induction technique
- Sterile anesthesia circuit is necessary for a portion of the procedure

Preparation

- Direct laryngoscopy and rigid bronchoscopy to evaluate severity of subglottic stenosis, its relative location to the vocal cords and to size the airway
- Airway sizing is done with an uncuffed ETT. The age-appropriate ETT is determined by using the following formula: (age + 16)/4. A leak test to 20 cm H_2O pressure is used to determine accurate size. For example, a 4-year-old child's airway should safely accommodate a 5.0 ETT.
- Effective neck extension is necessary using a shoulder roll
- A bougie esophageal dilator is placed before operation to allow for identification of the esophagus during elevation of the posterior trachea
- Preoperative discussion with family about possible conversion from CTR to LTR
- Chest prepped in the case of LTR conversion

Procedure

- Transverse cervical skin incision over the cricoid. Center around the tracheostomy stoma if planning single-stage surgery.
- This may be a double-staged procedure; however, there must be at least two normal tracheal rings between the tracheotomy site and the stenosis. If not, the tracheotomy should be included in the resection.
- Elevate skin flaps in the subcutaneous plane superiorly to the thyroid notch and inferiorly to the level of obstruction
- Gelpi retractors are placed
- Divide strap muscles and retract using 4-0 nonabsorbable monofilament sutures Skeletonize the thyroid cartilage and upper trachea. If the thyroid isthmus is encountered, it may be divided using cautery.
- Place 4-0 nonabsorbable monofilament sutures into the trachea inferior to the tracheotomy to gain positive control of the distal airway
- Place 4-0 nonabsorbable monofilament sutures on either side of the proposed vertical cricoid split
- A suprahyoid muscular release is performed to enable the laryngeal skeleton to become more mobile
- Mulliken and Grillo [11] found the average length of trachea that could be resected and

primarily anastomosed was 6.4 cm in the adult
larynx when releasing maneuvers were used

- In infants and children, Monnier et al. [10]
  have reported that resection of at least five
  tracheal rings is possible during CTR
- Wright et al. [12] performed a retrospective
  review of 116 children following tracheal surgery
  and found an average length of resected trachea
  of 3.4 cm and only 5.2% incidence of adjuvant
  tracheal release maneuver in this group
- Walner et al. [13] looked at their tracheal
  resection specimens following CTR in 38 children and found the longest length of resection
  was 3 cm
- A fine-tipped bipolar forceps is utilized to
  remove the cricothyroid muscle's medial
  attachment. This is tagged with a 4-0 monofilament suture for reapproximation at the end
  of the case.
- The theoretical advantage is vocal preservation
- A 6900 Beaver blade is utilized to vertically
  divide the anterior cricoid. A Jake hemostat is
  then utilized through the incision to distract
  the cricoid split. The incision is then carried
  superiorly to the thyroid cartilage and inferiorly
  to the first tracheal ring.
- The extent of the stenosis is then evaluated
  under direct vision
- If the stenosis is involving the first few tracheal
  rings, then they are divided as well
- If the subglottic stenosis is indistinct from the
  vocal cords, the CTR procedure is abandoned
  and a formal LTR is performed
- The cricoid is dissected free of the adjacent
  tissue in a subperichondrial plane in order to
  protect the recurrent laryngeal nerve. It is then
  removed in a piecemeal fashion laterally to the
  3 and 9 o'clock positions (fig. 1)
- The posterior cricoid mucosa is then elevated
  off the posterior cricoid using fine-tipped
  bipolar forceps and a Freer elevator. Prior to
  elevation, a tuberculin syringe with 27-gauge
  needle is then used to infiltrate the posterior
  cricoid mucosa with 1% lidocaine with

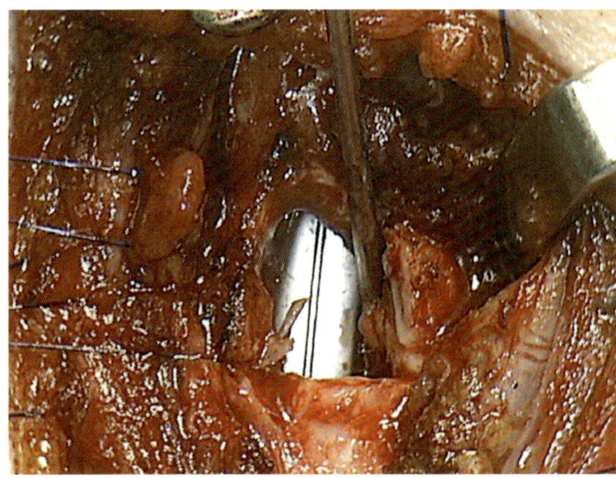

Fig. 1. Resection of the anterior cricoid in a piecemeal
fashion.

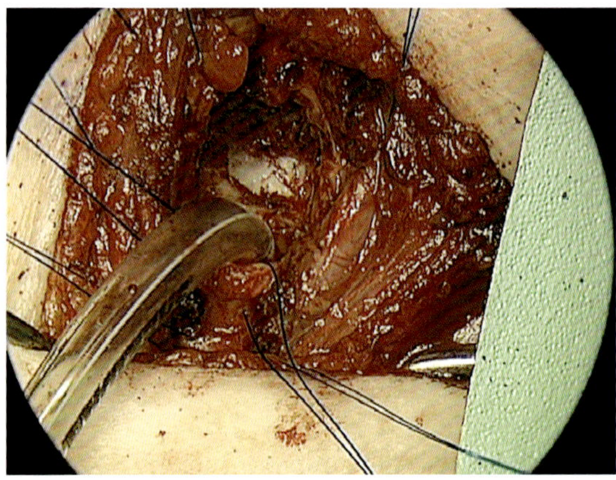

Fig. 2. Anterior cricoid has been resected, and posterior
cricoid is visible after it has been drilled down.

1:100,000 epinephrine. Less than 0.5 ml is
usually needed.

- An otologic drill with a 4-mm diamond burr is
  used to remove the cricoid ring laterally and to
  thin it posteriorly
- Take care to completely drill down the lateral
  walls so that there is a flat posterior plate with
  no lateral shelves remaining (fig. 2)
- Remove the tracheal rings involved in the
  stenosis

- The most superior uninvolved ring will be sacrificed in order to utilize its posterior mucosa for reanastomosis. This inferiorly based flap will cover the remaining thinned, posterior cricoid cartilage.
- Release the proximal tracheal rings from surrounding tissue using fine-tipped bipolar forceps in order to mobilize the distal trachea superiorly. This should be done anteriorly and laterally more than posteriorly in order to avoid devascularization of the trachea.
- Inferiorly, ensure that there are at least two strong and viable tracheal rings between the distal tracheal stump and the tracheal stoma (if a previous tracheotomy is in place). If not, include the stoma in the incision.
- Remove the shoulder roll
- Place 2-0 monofilament sutures inferiorly through the most proximal tracheal ring (submucosal) along the lateral aspect of the ring and through the thyroid cartilage superiorly. Pull together to assess for tension but do not tie at this time.
- Intubate from above in preparation for reanastomosis (if tracheotomy is removed)
- Nasotracheal: if there seems to be excessive tension on the anastomosis
- Orotracheal: if there seems to be appropriate tension of the anastomosis and postoperative extubation is possible
- Place 4-0 absorbable braided sutures to reapproximate the posterior mucosa of the most proximal tracheal ring to the mucosa overlying the posterior cricoid superiorly
- The posterior cricoid cartilage should be incorporated into this stitch (fig. 3, 4)
- An alternate suturing method directly reapproximates the mucosal flaps without incorporating the cricoid cartilage. This is performed if there is adequate superior mucosa (fig. 5).
- All posterior sutures should be thrown in an interrupted fashion. Tie these sutures only after all have been thrown.

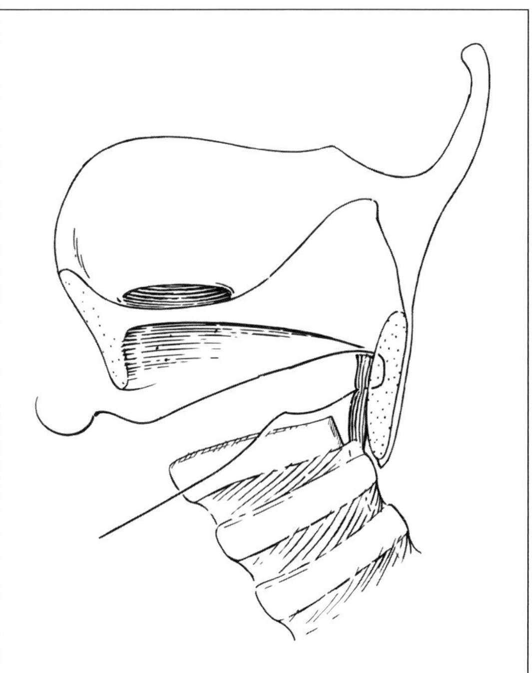

Fig. 3. Posterior anastomosis (lateral view).

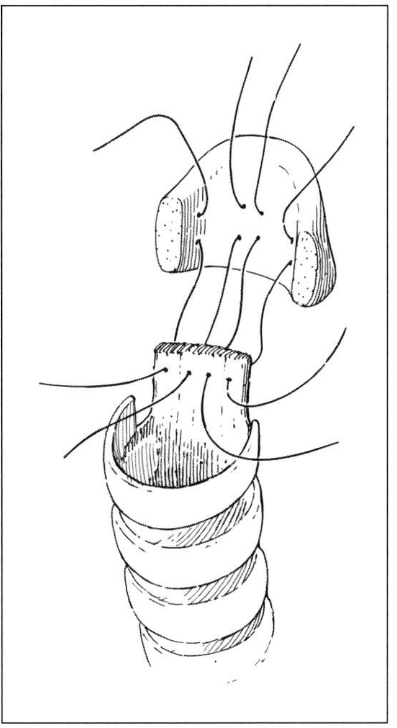

Fig. 4. Posterior anastomosis (anterior view).

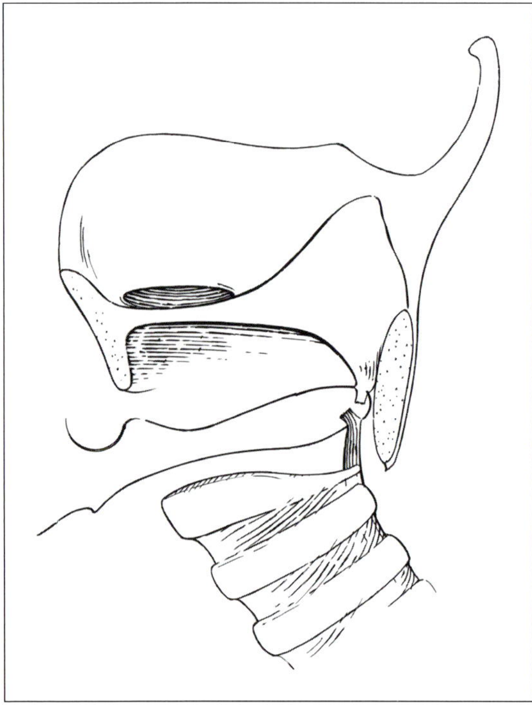

Fig. 5. Posterior anastomosis, variation.

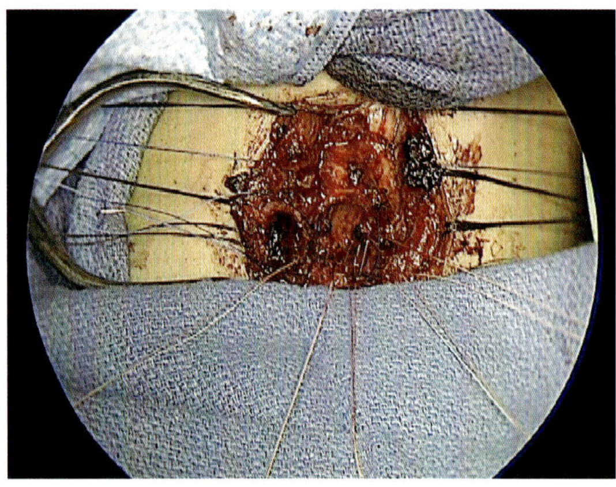

Fig. 6. Arranging the thrown sutures onto a clean blue towel prior to tying.

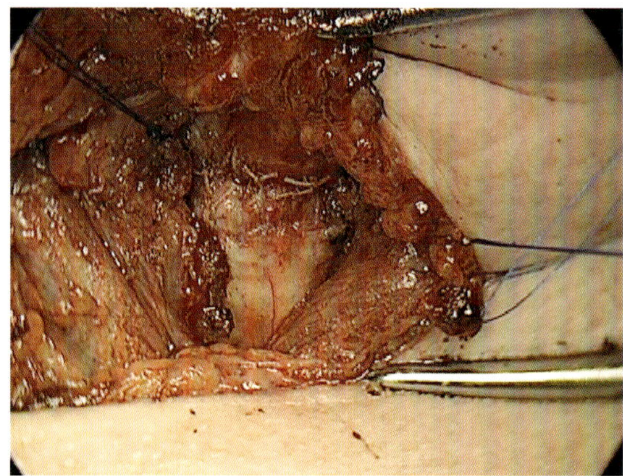

Fig. 7. Anterior trachea has been reapproximated and suture line is visible.

- Organizing all thrown/hemostat-tagged sutures on a clean blue towel is helpful to avoid crossing of suture lines (fig. 6)
- The 2-0 monofilament tension sutures described above are tied next
- The anterior mucosa is reapproximated using 4-0 absorbable braided suture. These should be interrupted and extraluminal. Again, all sutures should be thrown prior to tying (fig. 7–9).
- The cricothyroid muscle is reapproximated using 4-0 absorbable, braided sutures
- The wound is closed in a layered fashion. Fibrin glue sealant is placed over the trachea prior to closure of the strap muscles. A rubber band or Penrose drain is utilized for prevention of subcutaneous emphysema and hematoma/seroma formation.
- O monofilament chin-to-chest sutures are placed to keep the head from extending (fig. 10)

Postoperative Care

- Depending on the age/cooperation of the patient and the tension of the anastomosis, the patient may be extubated and placed in

Gallagher · Hartnick

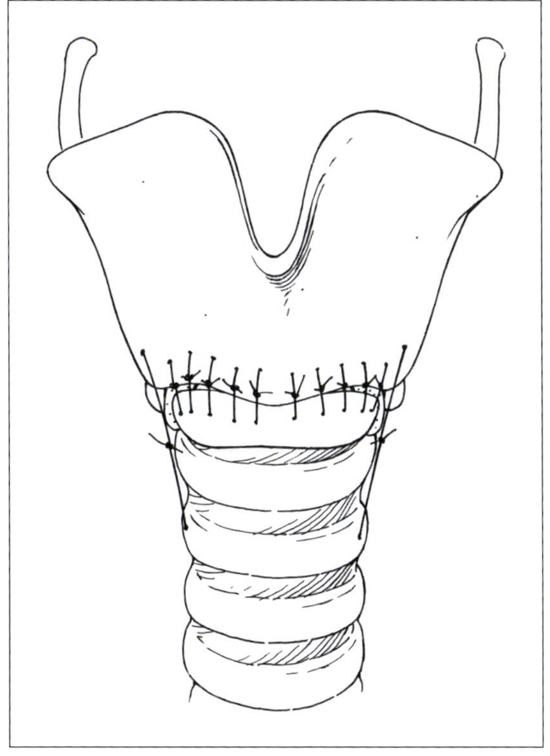

Fig. 8. Anterior anastomosis, anterior view.

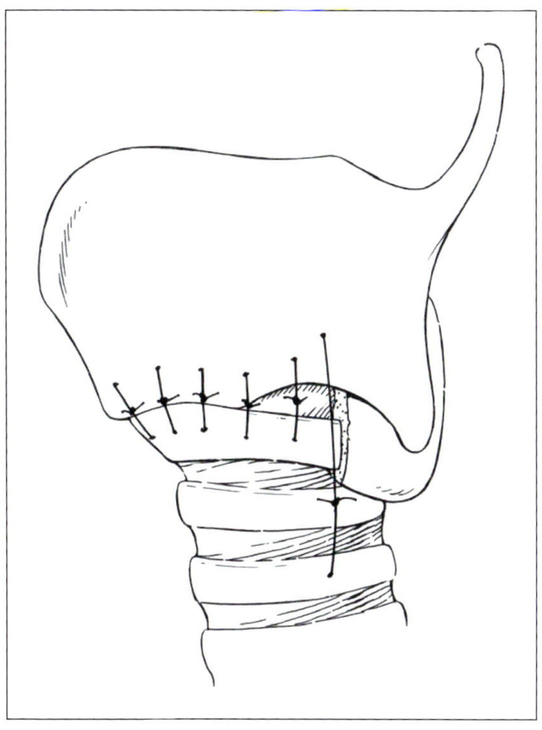

Fig. 9. Anterior anastomosis, lateral view. Note the mono-filament lateral suture spanning the anastomosis.

the PICU. Otherwise analgesia, sedation, and sometimes paralysis are necessary for patient immobilization.

- Prophylactic broad-spectrum intravenous antibiotics are given for 7 days
- Empiric proton pump inhibitor therapy for 3 months
- No i.v. steroids as this may inhibit critical wound healing
- Flexible fiber-optic laryngoscopy is performed to assess vocal fold mobility on postoperative day one (if extubated)
- Modified barium swallow is performed when patient is able to participate to determine aspiration risk prior to resuming oral diet
- Subcutaneous air must be assessed in the first few postoperative days. If it is present and

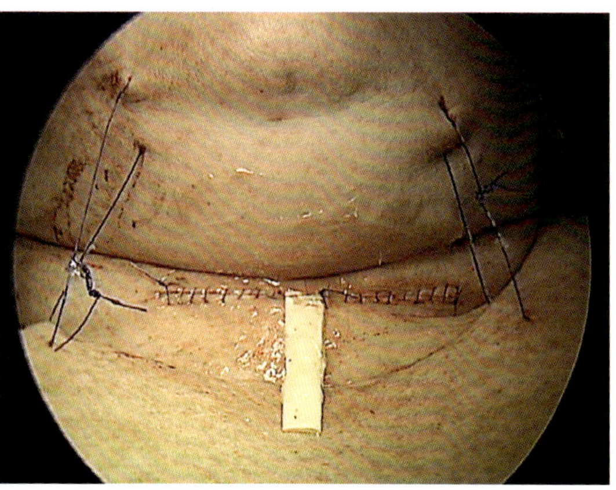

Fig. 10. Chin-to-chest sutures placed at the end of the case.

increasing, patient must be reintubated in the OR to prevent complications related to healing of the anastomosis.
- Repeat direct laryngoscopy and rigid bronchoscopy one week after surgery (do not balloon dilate at this time)

Pearls

- Bougie esophageal dilator placed preoperatively for easy identification of the esophagus
- Keep 4-0 retraction sutures organized so that any sutures retracting the airway are identifiable. In our OR, we use cut pieces of the magnetic instrument pad to separate muscle retraction sutures from airway retraction sutures.
- Retraction sutures on the distal trachea are essential in order to maintain adequate control of the airway during the procedure
- The recurrent laryngeal nerves are not identified. Careful subperichondrial dissection prevents damage to these structures.
- Use tuberculin syringe to palpate and gauge the depth of scar prior to posterior cricoid mucosa/scar elevation
- Remove the shoulder roll prior to reanastomosis
- The chin-to-chest sutures should allow the head to remain in neutral position and prevent extension. Maintenance of the head in a flexion position is not recommended.
- Just enough tension on the sutures so the head stays in a neutral, flex, or rotated position

Case Presentation

A 15-month-old male, former term infant, with a history of grade III subglottic stenosis presented with >10 episodes of recurrent croup and biphasic stridor. Direct laryngoscopy/tracheoscopy revealed grade III subglottic stenosis (fig. 11). It was decided to perform a tracheotomy based on his clinical presentation and endoscopic

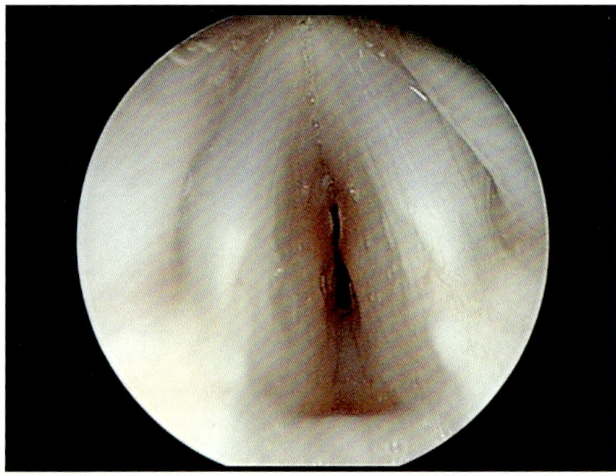

Fig. 11. Preoperative bronchoscopy.

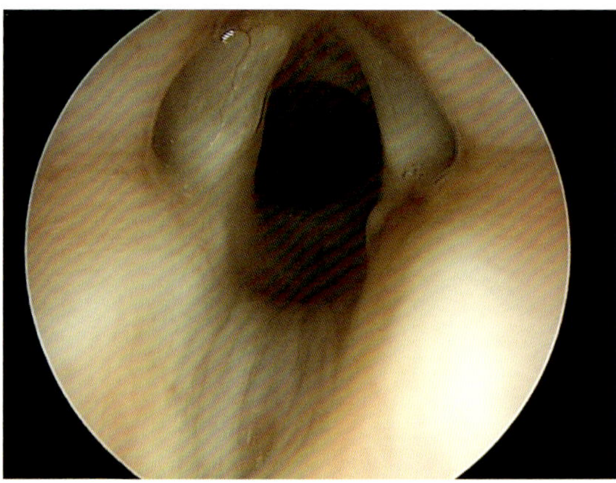

Fig. 12. Three years after operation.

evaluation. An LTR was performed with an anterior/posterior costal cartilage graft in a double-stage fashion using a #6 T-tube. In the following weeks, he developed a grade IV subglottic stenosis despite endoscopic interventions. A CTR was then performed 2 months later. The patient had an uneventful recovery with resolution of his stridor and was eventually decannulated (fig. 12).

References

1 Bath A, Panarese A, Thevagayam M, et al: Pediatric subglottic stenosis. Clin Otolaryngol 1999;24:117–121.

2 Berkowitz N, Oyos T, Murray D, et al: Postoperative care following single-stage laryngotracheoplasty. Ann Otol Rhinol Laryngol 1996;105:317–322.

3 Cotton R: The problem of pediatric laryngotracheal stenosis: a clinical and experimental study on the efficacy of autogenous cartilaginous grafts placed between vertically divided halves of the posterior lamina of the cricoid cartilage. Laryngoscope 1991;101:1–34.

4 Narcy P, Contencin P, Fligny I, et al: Surgical treatment for laryngotracheal stenosis in the pediatric patient. Arch Otolaryngol Head Neck Surg 1990;116:1047–1050.

5 Preciado D, Zalzal G: Laryngeal and tracheal stents in children. Curr Opin Otolaryngol Head Neck Surg 2008;16:83–85.

6 Gerwat J, Bryce DP: The management of subglottic laryngeal stenosis by reconstruction and direct anastomosis. Laryngoscope 1974;84:940–957.

7 Monnier P, Lang F, Savary M: Partial cricotracheal resection for pediatric subglottic stenosis: a single institution's experience in 60 cases. Eur Arch Otolaryngol 2003;260:295–297.

8 Monnier P, Lang F, Savary M: Partial cricotracheal resection for pediatric subglottic stenosis: update on the Lausanne experience. Ann Otol Rhinol Laryngol 1998;107:961–297.

9 Monnier P, Lang F, Savary M: Cricotracheal resection for pediatric subglottic stenosis. Int J Pediatr Otolaryngol 1999;49:S283–S286.

10 Monnier P, Savary M, Chapuis G: Partial cricoid resection with primary tracheal anastomosis for subglottic stenosis in infants and children. Laryngoscope 1993;103:1273–1283.

11 Mulliken JB, Grillo HC: The limits of tracheal resection with primary anastomosis. J Thorac Cardiovasc Surg 1968;55:418–421.

12 Wright CD, Graham BB, Grillo HC, et al: Pediatric tracheal surgery. Ann Thorac Surg 2002;74:308–313.

13 Walner DL, Stern Y, Cotton RT: Margins of partial cricotracheal resection in children. Laryngoscope 1999;109:1607–1610.

Thomas Q. Gallagher
LCDR, MC, USN
Naval Medical Center Portsmouth
Department of Otolaryngology, Bldg 3, 4th Floor
620 John Paul Jones Circle
Portsmouth, VA 23708 (USA)
E-Mail thomasqgallagher@yahoo.com

Hartnick CJ, Hansen MC, Gallagher TQ (eds): Pediatric Airway Surgery. Adv Otorhinolaryngol. Basel, Karger, 2012, vol 73, pp 50–57

Tracheal Resection and Reanastomosis

Thomas Q. Gallagher[a] · Christopher J. Hartnick[b]

[a]LCDR, MC, USN, Department of Otolaryngology, Naval Medical Center Portsmouth, Portsmouth, Va., [b]Department of Otology and Laryngology, Massachusetts Eye & Ear Infirmary, Boston, Mass., USA

Abstract

Isolated short segment tracheal stenosis occurs in a relatively rare subpopulation of patients with laryngotracheal stenosis. Etiologies include both acquired and congenital, the most common being the acquired type. Management options include observation, endoscopic balloon dilation with or without CO_2 laser, stent placement and open airway surgery. In this chapter, we will discuss tracheal resection and reanastomosis with emphasis on surgical pearls for success.

Although occurring in a relatively rare subpopulation of patients with laryngotracheal stenosis, isolated tracheal stenosis is amenable to several different management options. They include observation, endoscopic balloon dilation with or without CO_2 laser, stent placement and open airway surgery. In this chapter, we will discuss tracheal resection and reanastomosis.

Similar to the discussion of subglottic stenosis in the preceding chapter, tracheal stenosis can

be acquired or congenital. The etiology of acquired tracheal stenosis includes blunt trauma, intubation trauma (specifically high cuff pressures), and tracheostomy-induced granulation and subsequent suprastomal collapse and stenosis. These lesions can occur anywhere along the course of the trachea depending on the etiology. Congenital tracheal stenosis is rare with its incidence estimated at 1 in 64,500 [1]. These congenital lesions although often less severe than the acquired type can be associated with gastrointestinal, pulmonary, and cardiovascular malformations. Congenital tracheal stenosis is classified into three different types: (1) generalized hypoplasia, (2) funnel-like stenosis, and (3) segmental stenosis (fig. 1).

Both acquired and congenital tracheal stenosis can involve short or long segments. Tracheal resection and reanastomosis is reserved for short segment stenosis, typically about 3 cm or less [2, 3]. Treatment of long segment tracheal stenosis is discussed in the Slide Tracheoplasty chapter later in this volume. In this chapter, the authors will discuss tracheal resection and reanastomosis with emphasis on surgical pearls for success.

Relevant Anatomy

For relevant anatomy, see chapter 1.

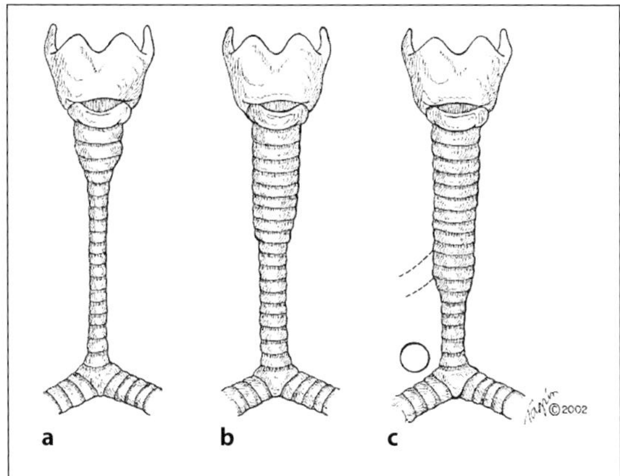

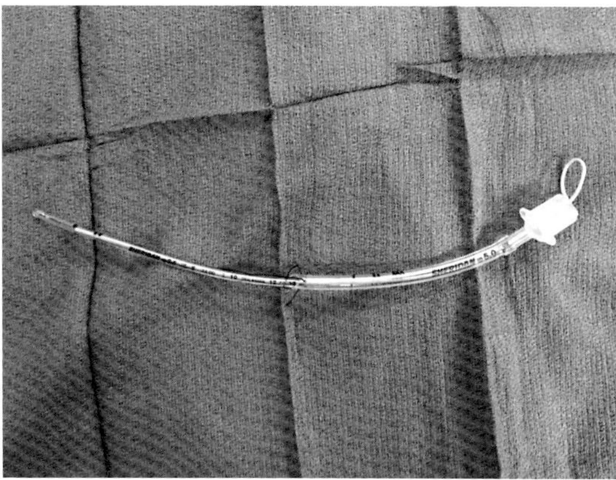

Fig. 1. General catagories of congenital tracheal stenosis. **a** Generalized hypoplasia. **b** Funnel-like stenosis. **c** Segmental stenosis. Reprinted with kind permission from Grillo HC: Surgery of the trachea and bronchi, BC Decker, 2004.

Fig. 2. Modifed endotracheal tube (ETT). This smaller diameter ETT is sutured to the end of a larger diameter ETT to effectively provide a long, narrow diameter ETT.

Indications

- Short-segment (<4–5 tracheal rings) congenital or acquired tracheal stenosis occluding >50% of the lumen
- Patients who have failed more conservative endoscopic interventions (i.e. laser and balloon dilation) for tracheal webs or stenosis
- Patients with symptomatic episodes of dyspnea on exertion, cyanosis, respiratory arrest, recurrent pulmonary infections
- Short-segment tracheomalacia not amenable to other treatment modalities (observation, BiPAP, tracheotomy, stent)

Contraindications

- Long-segment tracheal stenosis (defined as >5 tracheal rings)
- Uncontrolled gastroesophageal reflux or reactive airway disease
- Tracheostomy tube dependence due to chronic pulmonary disease or neurologic impairment

Anesthesia Considerations

- Communication is key
- May require cardiopulmonary bypass. ECMO is required for low tracheal lesions
- A modifed endotracheal tube (ETT) may be necessary as an emergency adjunct for distal stenosis in adolescents and adults. This smaller diameter ETT is sutured to the end of a larger diameter ETT to effectively provide a long, narrow-diameter ETT (fig. 2).
- It is helpful to have the patient spontaneously breathing at the time of reanastomosis to reduce intermittent intubation during aid placement of the posterior mucosal sutures

Preparation

- Preoperative:
- CT scan of neck and chest without contrast to measure airway (reconstructed images in plane with airway)
- Direct laryngoscopy and rigid bronchoscopy (DLB) to measure airway and compare with CT scan measurements

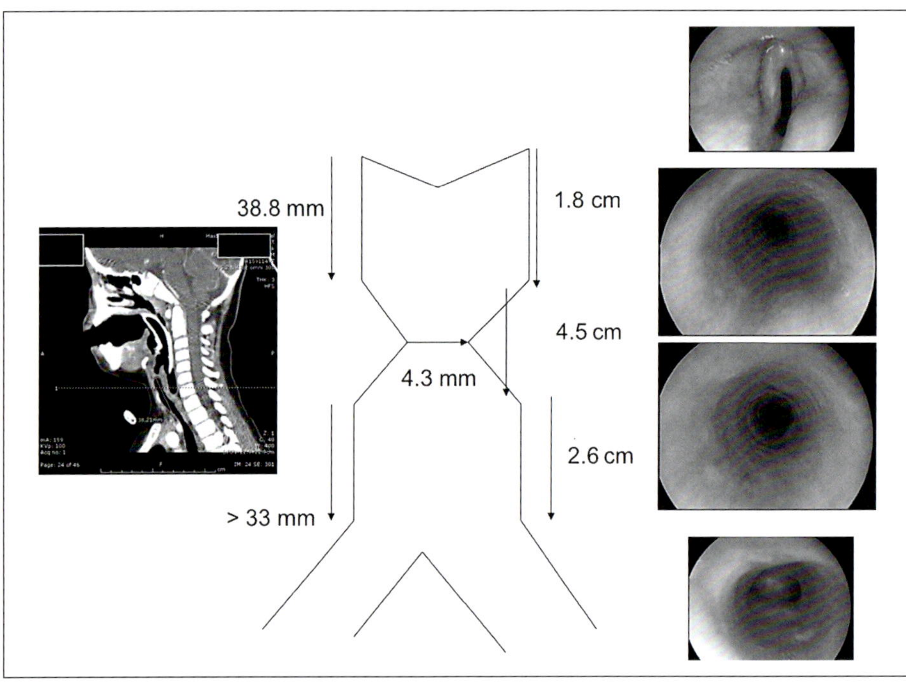

Fig. 3. "Roadmap" of the airway using CT scan and DLB measurements.

- Build 'roadmap' of the airway using CT scan and DLB measurements (fig. 3)
- Intraoperative:
- Generous shoulder roll for neck extension
- Repeat DLB to assess for any changes from preoperative DLB (i.e. inflammation)
- Skin prepped from chin to umbilicus
- If tracheostomy present, replace with cuffed endotracheal tube sutured to chest
- Appropriate-sized Bougie dilator into the esophagus to make the esophagus more prominent during dissection
- Local injection of lidocaine with 1:200,000 epinephrine at skin incision. This concentration is used in infants and young children.

Procedure

- Transverse cervical skin incision ellipsing the tracheotomy stoma (online suppl. video 1). If stoma is at least two tracheal rings clear of stenosis, then stoma would not be included in resection and would be removed separately.
- If no stoma is present, transverse incision is placed in prominent neck crease
- Subcutaneous flaps elevated from hyoid bone superiorly to below level of stenosis
- Strap muscles are divided and retracted with 4-0 Prolene sutures. The airway from hyoid to distal cervical trachea is exposed (fig. 4).
- Suprahyoid muscles are released from medial hyoid bone to allow for mobilization of the proximal trachea. This is facilitated using an Alice clamp for retraction (fig. 5).
- A small hypodermic needle is used to identify the stenosis externally, while a rigid bronchoscopy is performed to confirm the level of stenosis
- 4-0 Prolene retraction sutures are placed below the level of the stenosis to provide control of the distal airway

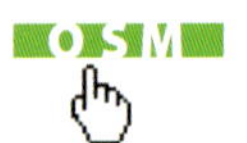

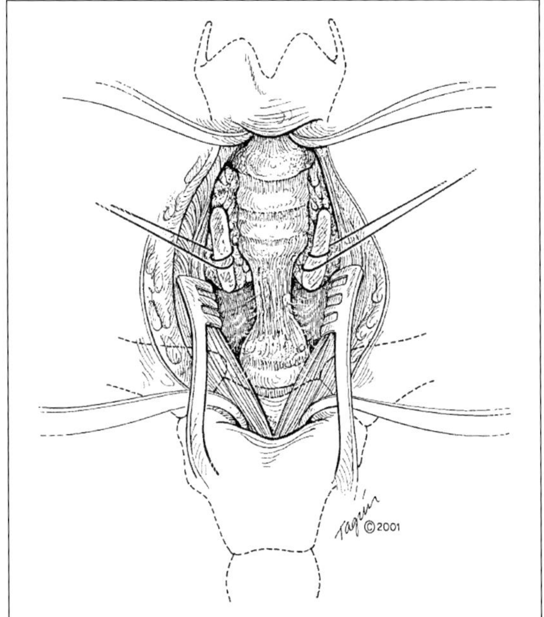

Fig. 4. Strap muscles are divided and retracted with 4-0 Prolene sutures. The airway from hyoid to distal cervical trachea is exposed demonstrating the area of stenosis. Reprinted with kind permission from Grillo HC: Surgery of the trachea and bronchi, BC Decker, 2004.

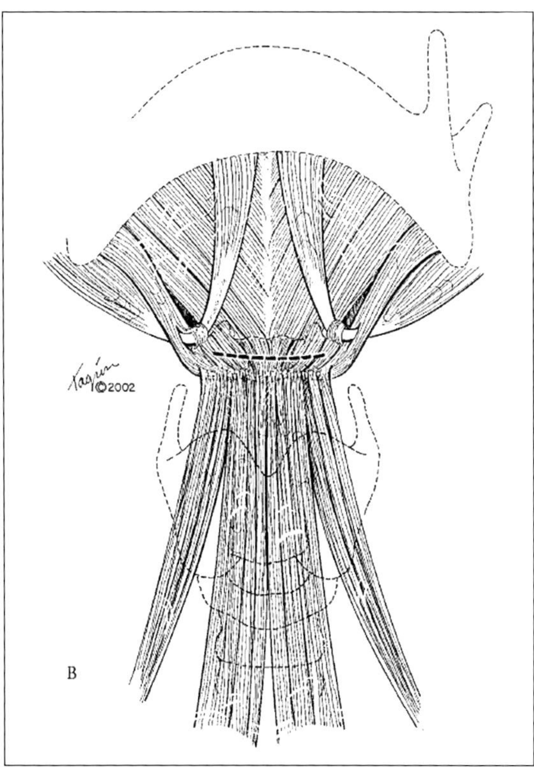

Fig. 5. Suprahyoid and infrahyoid muscle anatomy Reprinted with kind permission from Grillo HC: Surgery of the trachea and bronchi, BC Decker, 2004.

- The trachea is entered vertically with a 6900 Beaver blade, and the area of stenosis is inspected to determine the amount needed for resection. A vertically oriented incision allows easy closure if the surgery needs to be aborted (i.e. segment too long to resect).
- Piecemeal resection of the stenotic trachea is performed next. Direct visualization of the stenosis can be performed at this time to determine if stoma needs to be included with the stenosis. This is done if there are less than two tracheal rings between the stenosis and the stoma.
- Close dissection of the trachea is performed with sharp scissors or fine-tipped bipolar cautery. This dissection should occur in the sub-perichondrial plane. This close dissection is necessary to avoid damage to the recurrent laryngeal nerve. The nerves are not identified during the dissection.

- At this point, the endotracheal tube is withdrawn and the patient is intubated through the distal tracheal segment (fig. 6)
- Replace endotracheal tube intermittently to perform dissection of posterior stenosis. It is important to have the patient spontaneously breathing at this point to allow for long periods without the patient intubated.
- Elevation of the soft tissues from the anterior and lateral distal trachea enable mobilization of this segment
- Removal of the shoulder roll at this point of the surgery will help with reapproximation of the distal and proximal segments
- 2-0 Prolene sutures are placed (but not tied) at the 3 and 9 o'clock positions of the trachea in a

submucosal fashion. Ensure this suture spans at least two complete rings in order for it to provide a significant hold. If there is too much tension on the anastomosis, the patient will be nasotracheally intubated postoperatively for several days. If the tension is not deemed significant, then the patient may be extubated provided he/she can keep his/her head in the appropriate position.

- Reanastomosis of the posterior trachea is done with 4-0 vicryl sutures in a buried, extra-luminal fashion. Five sutures in total are thrown starting from midline and working laterally. Sutures are not tied until all are thrown (fig. 7).
- The patient is then intubated orally
- The anterior trachea is then sutured using 4-0 vicryl in a simple, interrupted fashion using five sutures in total. Sutures may be intraluminal, and are not tied until all the sutures are thrown. The 2-0 Prolene 'tension' sutures are tied at this point (fig. 8).
- The wound is closed in a layered fashion. Fibrin glue sealant is placed over the trachea prior to closure of the strap muscles. A Penrose drain is utilized for prevention of subcutaneous emphysema.

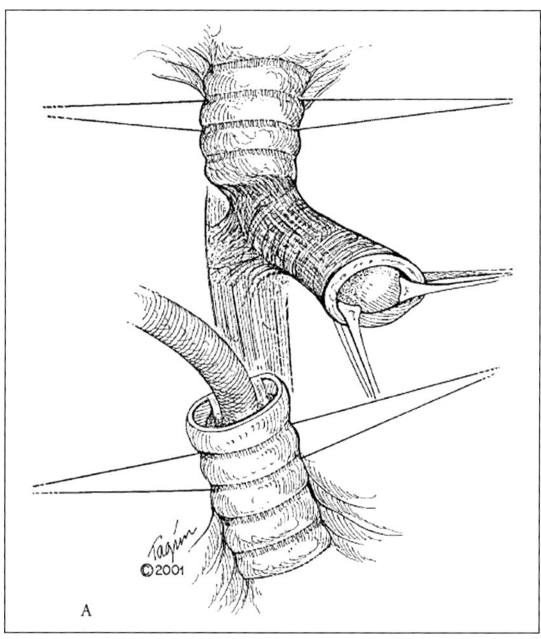

Fig. 6. The proximal and distal segments are demonstrated. The ETT is withdrawn and the patient is intubated through the distal tracheal segment. Reprinted with kind permission from Grillo HC: Surgery of the trachea and bronchi, BC Decker, 2004.

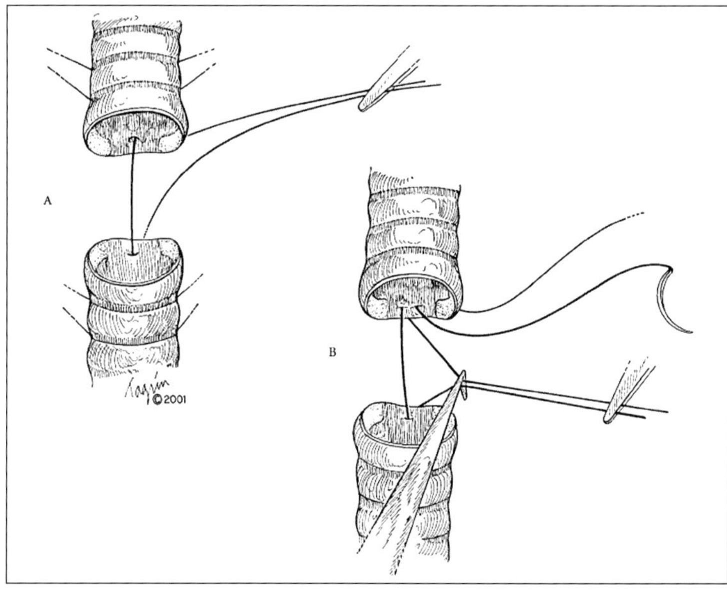

Fig. 7. Re-anastomosis of the trachea is done with 4-0 Vicryl sutures in a buried, extra-luminal fashion. Five sutures total are thrown starting from midline and working laterally. No sutures are not tied until all are thrown. Reprinted with kind permission from Grillo HC: Surgery of the trachea and bronchi, BC Decker, 2004.

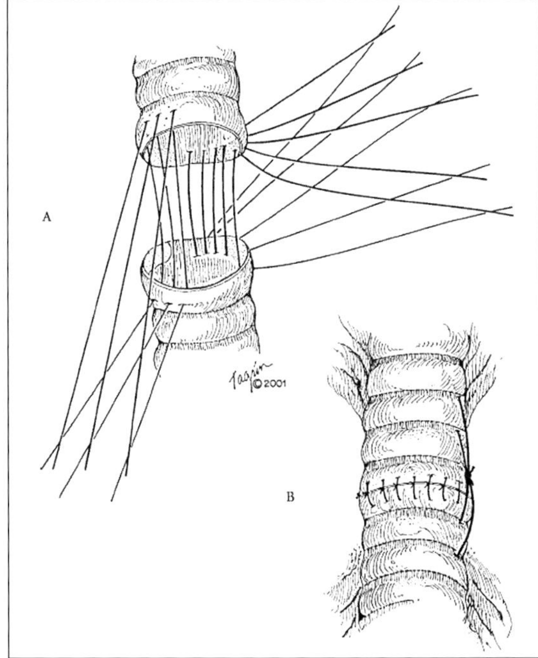

Fig. 8. a The anterior trachea is then sutured using 4-0 Vicryl in a simple, interrupted fashion using approximately five sutures total. **b** The 2-0 Prolene "tension" sutures are tied at this point (lateral trachea). Reprinted with kind permission from Grillo HC: Surgery of the trachea and bronchi, BC Decker, 2004.

- 0 Prolene chin-chest sutures are thrown bilaterally. The sutures should allow the head to rest easily in the neutral position.

Postoperative Care

- Depending on the age/cooperation of the patient and the tension of the anastomosis, the patient may be extubated and placed in the PICU. Otherwise analgesia, sedation, and sometimes paralysis are necessary for patient immobilization.
- Prophylactic intravenous antibiotics are given for 7 days
- Empiric proton pump inhibitor therapy for 3 months
- No i.v. steroids

- Flexible fiber-optic laryngoscopy is performed to assess vocal fold mobility on postoperative day one
- Modified barium swallow is performed when patient is able to participate to determine aspiration risk prior to resuming oral diet
- Subcutaneous air must be assessed in the first few postoperative days. If it is present and increasing, patient must be reintubated in the OR to prevent complications related to healing of the anastomosis.
- Repeat DLB one week after surgery (do not balloon dilate at this time)

Pearls

- Communication with anesthesia to have the patient spontaneously breathing for the reanastomosis
- Elevation of soft tissues from the anterior and lateral distal trachea enables mobilization of this segment. Take care not to dissect esophagus off the distal trachea, as this will jeopardize the blood supply to the trachea.
- Ensure to take the shoulder roll out to assist with tension-free closure. Excess tension can lead to mucosal separation, scaring and restenosis.
- Penrose drain to prevent subcutaneous emphysema
- Different release mobilization techniques include: Relan maneuver, suprahyoid release, annular ligament release, and bronchial release

Case Presentation

A 16-year-old otherwise healthy male was involved in a motor vehicle accident 7 months before. He was intubated for 8 days and had significant orthopedic, thoracic and abdominal injuries requiring prolonged hospitalization. After discharge from the hospital, he developed significant expiratory stridor and severe airway limitations. His

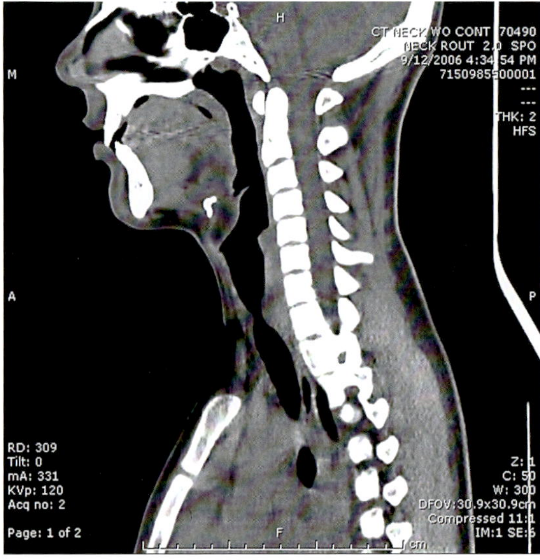

Fig. 9. A CT scan reveals concentric cervical tracheal stenosis about 1–2 cm in length.

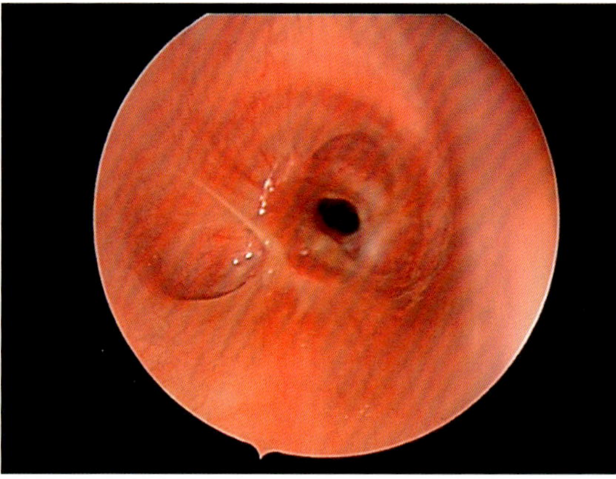

Fig. 11. A close-up view of figure 10 demonstrating significant, concentric tracheal stenosis.

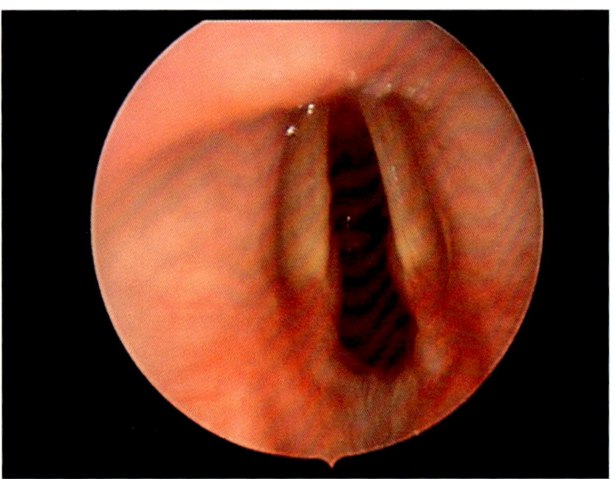

Fig. 10. A direct laryngoscopy/bronchoscopy demonstrated significant, concentric stenosis.

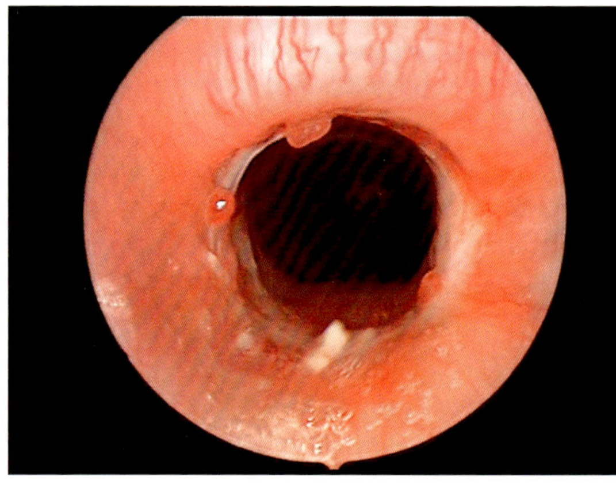

Fig. 12. One month post-operative tracheoscopy.

physical exam revealed audible expiratory stridor, and his flexible fiber-optic nasolaryngoscopy revealed bilateral vocal cord mobility. A CT scan of his chest revealed concentric tracheal stenosis of the cervical trachea just below the thyroid cartilage measuring about 1–2 cm in length (fig. 9). A direct laryngoscopy/bronchoscopy demonstrated significant, concentric stenosis (fig. 10, 11). After much discussion with the patient and family, tracheal resection and reanastomosis were decided upon over more conservative laser/balloon dilation. The surgery was performed, and his postoperative course was uneventful. His 1-month postoperative tracheoscopy is shown in figure 12.

Gallagher · Hartnick

References

1 Herrera P, Caldarone C, Forte V, et al: The current state of congenital tracheal stenosis. Pediatr Surg Int 2007;23:1033–1044.

2 Wright CD, Graham BB, Grillo HC, et al: Pediatric tracheal surgery. Ann Thorac Surg 2002;74:308–313.

3 Walner DL, Stern Y, Cotton RT: Margins of partial cricotracheal resection in children. Laryngoscope 1999;109:1607–1610.

Christopher J. Hartnick, MD
Professor, Department of Otology and Laryngology
Chief, Division of Pediatric Otolaryngology
Director, Pediatric Airway, Voice and Swallowing Center
Chief Quality Officer
Massachusetts Eye and Ear Infirmary, Harvard Medical School
243 Charles Street
Boston, MA 02116 (USA)
E-Mail christopher_hartnick@meei.harvard.edu

Hartnick CJ, Hansen MC, Gallagher TQ (eds): Pediatric Airway Surgery. Adv Otorhinolaryngol. Basel, Karger, 2012, vol 73, pp 58–62

Slide Tracheoplasty

Thomas Q. Gallagher[a] · Christopher J. Hartnick[b]

[a]LCDR, MC, USN, Department of Otolaryngology, Naval Medical Center Portsmouth, Portsmouth, Va., [b]Department of Otology and Laryngology, Massachusetts Eye & Ear Infirmary, Boston, Mass., USA

Abstract

Slide tracheoplasty, first described in 1989, has become the procedure of choice for long segment tracheal stenosis and complete tracheal rings. Although a challenging surgery with higher mortality than other open airway procedures, this technique offers a successful alternative for parents who just a couple decades ago had no reasonable surgical option. We describe the management of long segment tracheal stenosis using the slide tracheoplasty highlighting the surgical pearls necessary for success.

Long segment tracheal stenosis (LSTS) is a rare, life-threatening, usually congenital disorder. Children usually present with anything from simple stridor to near-death episodes at home sometimes requiring extracorporeal membrane oxygenation (ECMO) due to the inability to ventilate them [1]. LSTS is usually associated with congenital heart defects (pulmonary artery sling is one of the more common) and complete tracheal rings. As opposed to more common isolated airway stenoses (such as subglottic stenosis) that can be managed well with open airway surgery, LSTS is more challenging to manage and can be associated with higher mortality rates. The incorporation of ECMO and cardiopulmonary bypass (CPB) has helped reduce the mortality and allow for shorter operative time.

Although there exist several different techniques (costal cartilage tracheoplasty, pericardial patch tracheoplasty, tracheal resection, tracheal autograft tracheoplasty, and slide tracheoplasty) for management of infants and children with LSTS and congenital tracheal rings, slide tracheoplasty has emerged as the treatment of choice for this pathology [2]. It has been over the past 20 years that the slide tracheoplasty has become the mainstay of treatment for LSTS. It was first described by Tsang et al. [3] in 1989; Grillo et al. [4] later popularized it in the 1990s. Simply described, after dividing the stenotic segment at its midpoint, the upper and lower segments are incised vertically, and the corners trimmed in order to allow them to be sutured in an overlapping technique, which results in a shortening of the trachea but doubling of the airway diameter (fig. 1; online suppl. video 1). Macchiarini et al. [5] studied slide tracheoplasty in animals and noted the circumference of the trachea is doubled and the cross-sectional area quadrupled. They also noted subsequent tracheal growth was not

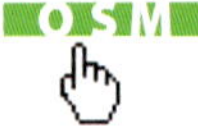

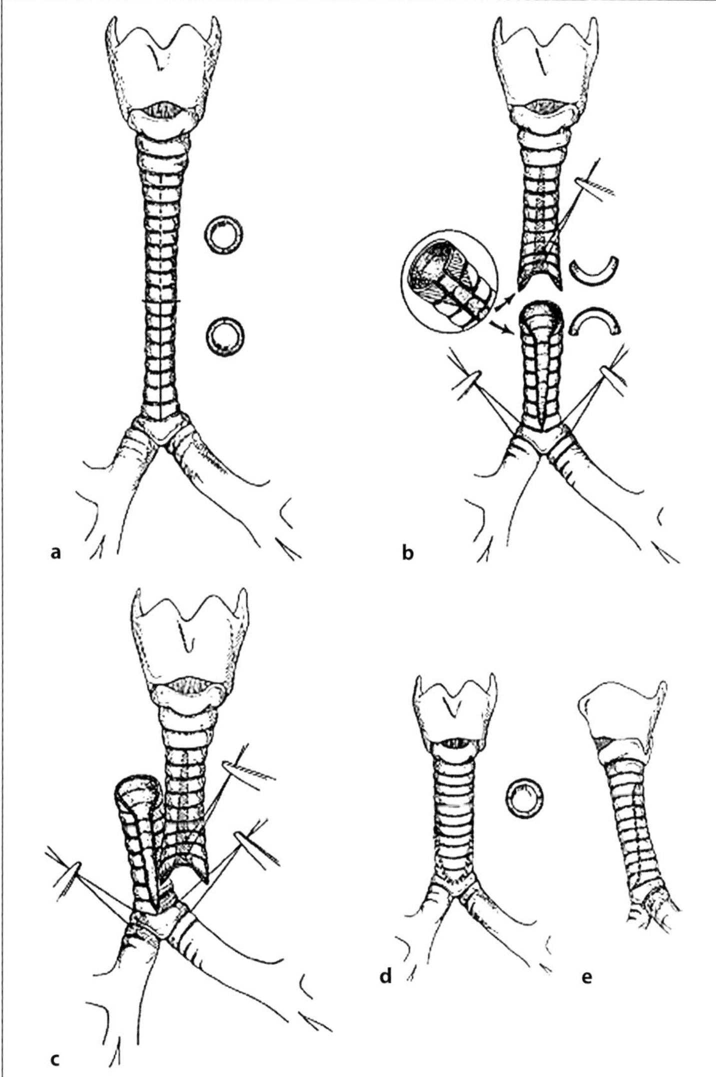

Fig. 1. Technique of slide tracheoplasty. **a** The extent of stenosis is identified precisely. The stenotic segment is divided transversely at its midpoint after circumferential dissection at that locus only. The upper stenotic segment is incised vertically posteriorly, and the lower segment anteriorly for the full length of the stenosis. **b** The right-angled corners produced by these divisions are trimmed above and below. A stay suture near the tip of the superior flap is helpful, as are traction sutures at the tracheobronchial angles or within the mainstem bronchi below. The 2 ends are slid together (**c**) after placement of individual anastomotic sutures around the entire oblique circumference of the tracheoplasty site (**d**, **e**). Reprinted with kind permission from Archives of Otolaryngology, 1998, 124:98–103. Copyright 1998, American Medical Association. All rights reserved.

inhibited. Additional benefits of the procedure include only native tissue is used, and normal ciliated respiratory epithelium is present immediately after surgery.

Anatomy

For anatomy, please refer to the section titled 'Adjacent Vascular and Cardiac Anomalies' in the Laryngeal Development and Anatomy chapter (pp. 1–11).

Indications

- LSTS (>2/3 of trachea)
- Complete tracheal rings almost always are found in patients that have LSTS
- This includes acquired LSTS

Contraindications

- Presence of a bronchus suis ('pig bronchus', see chapter 2 (pp 12–18)) with significant tracheal length between itself and the carina causes a problem with mobilization of the trachea
- This becomes an issue if there is distal LSTS; however, mid-tracheal LSTS may still be possible

Anesthesia Considerations

Although this procedure can be performed using conventional mechanical ventilation with the surgeon intermittently intubating during the procedure, it is significantly facilitated by ECMO or CPB.

Preparation

- Preoperative direct laryngoscopy and bronchoscopy are performed if possible
- The goal of this evaluation is to determine the length and width of the tracheal stenosis, the location of the most stenotic region whether or not there are any other associated airway anomalies (i.e. pulmonary sling, bronchus suis, etc.). Similar to the discussion in the chapter titled 'Tracheal Resection and Reanastomosis', a 'road-map' of the airway is created from the measurements obtained from bronchoscopy and CT.
- As with any bronchoscopy of a stenotic airway, erring on the side of caution during this evaluation is essential so one does not make a marginal airway a critical one due to swelling after the bronchoscopy
- In some cases, the preoperative bronchoscopy is abridged and the surgeon will need to perform intraoperative bronchoscopy to define the stenosis
- CT of the chest with contrast is helpful in determining approximate length of stenosis

and adjacent cardiac anatomy and possible anomalies
- Pulmonary artery sling is the most common type associated with LSTS
- Concomitant cardiac anomalies may be repaired simultaneously with the slide tracheoplasty
- Echocardiogram for evaluation of any cardiac anomalies
- CPB or ECMO:
- CPB is utilized if the distal third of the trachea is stenotic and if there is a concomitant cardiovascular lesion requiring thoracotomy for repair
- ECMO may be used for an isolated low or mid-segment slide tracheoplasty procedure where distal cannulation with an endotracheal tube or jet ventilation may not be feasible
- It is the senior author's preference to perform slide tracheoplasty under ECMO for procedures not requiring concomitant cardiac procedures, but the choice between ECMO and CPB may well be center and institution specific

Procedure

- Any cardiac repair is performed prior to the slide tracheoplasty
- A midline, low-cervical incision is marked out. This procedure is generally performed on very young children with long segment complete rings or stenosis as the first procedure where no previous tracheotomy has been performed or is possible. If a tracheotomy is present, the incision includes the stoma and is done as a single stage procedure.
- Appropriate-sized bougie dilator into the esophagus to make the esophagus more prominent during dissection
- Local injection of lidocaine with 1:200,000 epinephrine at skin incision. This concentration is used in infants and young children.

- Subcutaneous flaps elevated from hyoid bone superiorly to below level of stenosis
- Strap muscles are divided and retracted with 4-0 Prolene sutures. The airway from hyoid to distal cervical trachea is exposed.
- Suprahyoid muscles are released from medial hyoid bone to allow for mobilization of the proximal trachea. This is facilitated using an Alice clamp for retraction.
- The anterior tracheal is then exposed.
– The use of either ECMO or CPB greatly facilitates exposure of the stenotic segment because the innominate artery is retracted and brought away from the trachea thus exposing the entire distal trachea
- Use of a hypodermic needle and intraoperative bronchoscopy can be helpful in determining the exact location to transect the stenosis at its midpoint as well as determination of the length of the stenosis
– This is helpful in determining where to transect the trachea as well as how long to make the incisions in the proximal and distal segments
- The trachea is divided at the midpoint of the stenosis
- The end of the proximal and distal tracheal are mobilized
- The posterior wall of the proximal segment is incised superiorly for the length of the stenosis
- The anterior wall of the distal segment is incised inferiorly for the length of the stenosis or carina, whichever is encountered first. The reason for orienting these incisions in the proximal and distal segments is due to the fact that it would be far more difficult to access the posterior incision were it made in the distal segment.
- The distal ends of each segment are trimmed to facilitate closure
- The segments are then overlapped with the proximal segment placed anteriorly
- It is the senior author's preference to use interrupted 5-0 (infants and children) or 4-0 (adolescents) polyglactin sutures using Dr. Grillo's described technique [6], although other centers do describe the use of a running suture technique [2]
– Sutures are placed approximately 3 mm apart through the full thickness of the trachea so that the knots will be extraluminal
– Suturing is begun proximally and carried in parallel succession distally, the final suture being placed at the distal end of the anterior wall of the upper segment of the trachea
– All sutures are thrown before being tied
– Prior to closure of the trachea, the patient is nasotracheally intubated under direct vision
- Fibrin glue is placed over the trachea to assist with healing
- A leak test is performed by flooding the surgical field with saline solution and performing a Valsalva to 20 cm of water pressure
- The patient is taken off bypass or ECMO
- The chest is then closed by the cardiothoracic surgeon if CPB was employed
- The neck wound is then closed in a layered fashion over a passive drain
- Chin to chest sutures are placed to prevent inadvertent extension of the patient's head for the first week
- The bougie is removed and replaced with a nasogastric feeding tube

Postoperative Care

- Postoperative recovery in the pediatric intensive care unit
- The patient may either be extubated at the time of the procedure or left intubated for several days via nasotracheal intubation depending upon the surgeon's preference and the tension on the anastomosis
- A bronchoscopy is performed one week later
- It is the senior author's preference not to balloon before 6 weeks following this procedure

Pearls

- Abbreviated bronchoscopy if the risk of postbronchoscopy airway swelling is too great
- Use of ECMO when indicated and when either jet ventilation or distal endotracheal intubation would be difficult
- Maintaining the lateral vascular attachments of the proximal and distal tracheal segments
- CPB when additional cardiac procedures required
- It is the senior author's preference to use interrupted sutures for closure so as to protect against dehiscence were one suture to break and to help avoid the formation of the postoperative hourglass shape of the airway that can occur when only one suture is used for closure and it is tightly drawn

References

1 Elliott M, Roebuck D, Noctor C, et al: The management of congenital tracheal stenosis. Int J Pediatr Otorhinolaryngol 2003;67(suppl 1):S183–S192.
2 Rutter MJ, Cotton RT, Azizkhan, Manning PB: Slide tracheoplasty for the management of complete tracheal rings. J Pediatr Surg 2003;38:928–934.
3 Tsang V, Murday A, Gilbe C, et al: Slide tracheoplasty for congenital funnel shaped tracheal stenosis. Ann Thorac Surg 1989;48:632–635.
4 Grillo HC, Wright CD, Vlahakes GJ, et al: Management of congenital tracheal stenosis by means of slide tracheoplasty or resection and reconstruction, with long-term follow-up of growth after slide tracheoplasty. J Thorac Cardiovasc Surg 2002;123:145–152.
5 Macchiarini P, Dulmet E, de Montpreville V, et al: Tracheal growth after slide tracheoplasty. J Thorac Cardiovasc Surg 1997;113:558–566.
6 Cunningham MJ, Eavey RD, Vlahakes GJ, Grillo HC: Slide tracheoplasty for long segment tracheal stenosis. Arch Otolaryngol Head Neck Surg 1998;124:98–103.

Christopher J. Hartnick, MD
Professor, Department of Otology and Laryngology
Chief, Division of Pediatric Otolaryngology
Director, Pediatric Airway, Voice and Swallowing Center
Chief Quality Officer
Massachusetts Eye and Ear Infirmary, Harvard Medical School
243 Charles Street
Boston, MA 02116 (USA)
E-Mail christopher_hartnick@meei.harvard.edu

Hartnick CJ, Hansen MC, Gallagher TQ (eds): Pediatric Airway Surgery. Adv Otorhinolaryngol. Basel, Karger, 2012, vol 73, pp 63–65

Suprastomal Granuloma

Thomas Q. Gallagher[a] · Christopher J. Hartnick[b]

[a]LCDR, MC, USN, Department of Otolaryngology, Naval Medical Center Portsmouth, Portsmouth, Va., [b]Department of Otology and Laryngology, Massachusetts Eye & Ear Infirmary, Boston, Mass., USA

Abstract

Suprastomal granuloma is one of the most common sequelae of pediatric tracheotomy. Numerous different techniques have been described for their removal including endoscopic and open procedures. The following chapter discusses the intraoperative techniques for open removal of suprastomal granuloma in infants.

One of the most common complications of pediatric tracheotomy is formation of a suprastomal granuloma (SSG). This has been reported in anywhere from 4 to 80% of pediatric tracheotomies, and based on its frequency some authors question if it truly represents a complication [1–3]. The etiology of SSG formation is unknown but may represent trauma from the initial procedure, pooling of secretions, or chronic infection [4]. Additionally, there has been no described method to prevent SSG formation.

Surveillance for and management of SSG varies from surgeon to surgeon. The authors' preference for SSG surveillance includes a direct laryngoscopy

and rigid tracheoscopy every 6 months in children less than 2 years of age. Additionally, any significant bleeding from the tracheostomy tube or difficulty with tracheostomy tube changes warrants an evaluation under anesthesia. A recent survey of ASPO members in 2011 regarding management techniques for SSG included skin hook and eversion (68%), microdebrider (35%), and laser (14%) [5]. Other techniques described include optical forceps [6], sphenoid punch [7], and coblation [8].

In this chapter, we will discuss the open management of SSG. We perform this technique in infants who have a tracheotomy and the granuloma is either too large for the above-stated techniques or the airway is too small to accommodate an endoscopic approach for removal.

Indications

- Large obstructing SSG that meets the following conditions:
- Too large or firm (mature) to remove via endoscopic techniques
- Too large or firm (mature) to remove via the stoma

Anesthesia Considerations

- Open dialogue and communication with anesthesia

- Induction using general inhalation anesthesia via tracheostomy tube
- Changing to an endotracheal tube placed through the tracheostoma is done after induction
- Maintaining low oxygen settings during use of electrocautery to reduce the risk of airway fire
- Replacing the tracheostomy tube after completion of the procedure

Preparation

- Prior to the open neck procedure, a direct laryngoscopy and rigid tracheoscopy should be performed to evaluate the airway. Figure 1 shows a large SSG 100% obstructing the airway (see also online suppl. video 1).
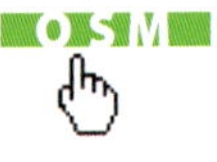
- Generous shoulder roll and neck extension for exposure
- Povidone-iodine skin preparation after replacement of the tracheostomy tube with an age appropriate endotracheal tube

Procedure

- The neck is marked with a small, 2- to 3-cm incision just superior to the tracheostoma. It is injected with 1% lidocaine with 1:100,000 epinephrine.
- The incision is made and dissection continues down through the soft tissue. The strap muscles are divided and the trachea is identified.
  - It is important to stay superior to the stoma tract. Violation of the tract has the potential for false passage creation postoperatively similar to what can occur after a fresh tracheotomy.
  - If the thyroid is encountered, it is divided in the midline with electrocautery
- The trachea is then opened in the midline with a small vertical incision. Usually, this is at the level of the second or first tracheal ring.
  - Care is taken to avoid accidental division of the cricoid

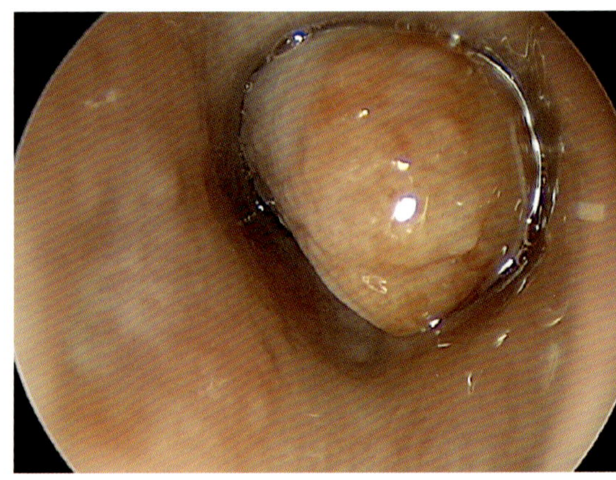

Fig. 1. Endoscopic view of a large suprastomal granuloma obstructing 100% of the airway.

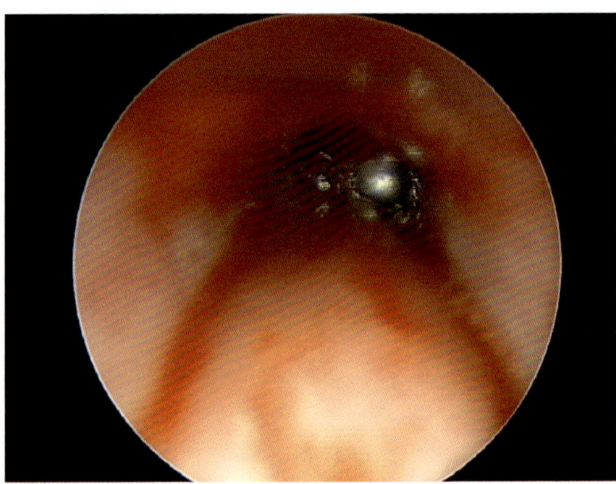

Fig. 2. Post-operative endoscopic view after open removal of obstructing suprastomal granuloma.

- The granuloma is identified and can be grasped with a fine hemostat or right-angled clamp. A small, fine scissor or scalpel is then used to remove the granuloma.
- The airway is then reevaluated to ensure complete removal (fig. 2). Sometimes, performing a direct laryngoscopy/tracheoscopy with a Hopkins rod-lens telescope can assist with this evaluation.
- The airway is then closed using 3-0 braided, absorbable suture placed in a simple interrupted fashion. Care is taken to throw these sutures extra-luminally.
- Fibrin sealant is then applied

Gallagher · Hartnick

- The wound is then closed in a layered fashion over a passive drain to allow for air escape and to help prevent possible formation of subcutaneous air (fig. 3)
- The tracheostomy tube is replaced

Postoperative Care

- A chest X-ray is obtained in the postoperative anesthesia care unit to ensure there is no pneumothorax
- The patient is observed overnight and the drain is removed on the first postoperative day provided there is no subcutaneous air formation
- A suture removal kit is left at the bedside and the call team is instructed on its use in the unlikely case of expanding subcutaneous emphysema causing airway compromise
- The parents are instructed to resume regular tracheostomy tube changes in one week

Pearls

- Preoperative direct laryngoscopy/tracheoscopy is essential to understand the airway anatomy

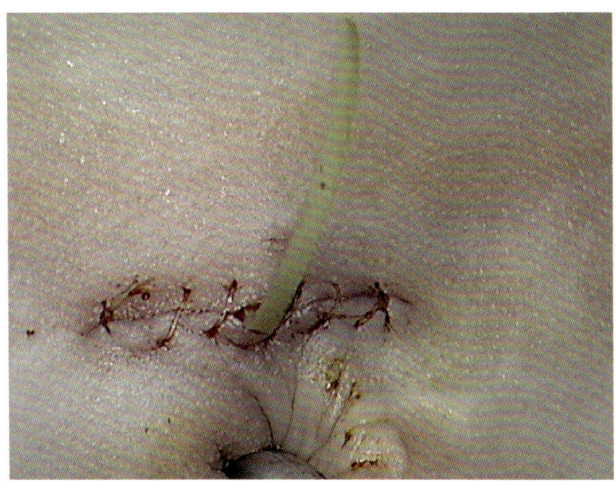

Fig. 3. A post-operative view of the incision with passive drain in place.

- Exposure of the airway and identification of normal landmarks is important to avoid inadvertent damage to the cricoid when opening the trachea
- Care must be taken not to violate the mature stoma tract during dissection as this could lead to possible complications when replacing the tracheostomy tube if there is accidental decannulation in the immediate postoperative time period

References

1 Rosenfield RM, Stool SE: Should granulomas be excised in children with long-term tracheotomy? Arch Otolaryngol Head Neck Surg 1992;118:1323–1327.
2 Tom LW, Miller L, Wetmore RF, et al: Endoscopic assessment of children with tracheotomies. Arch Otolaryngol Head Neck Surg 1993;119:321–324.
3 Reilly JS, Myer CM: Excision of suprastomal granulation tissue. Laryngoscope 1985;95:1545–1546.
4 Rodgers JH: Decannulation by external exploration of the tracheostomy in children. J Laryngol Otol 1980;94:563–567.
5 Kraft S, Patel S, Sykes K, et al: Practice patterns after tracheotomy in infants younger than 2 years. Arch Otolaryngol Head Neck Surg 2011;137:670–674.
6 Yellon RF: Totally obstructing tracheotomy-associated suprastomal granulation tissue. Int J Pediatr Otorhinolaryngol 2000;53:49–55.
7 Prescott CAJ: Peristomal complications of paediatric tracheostomy. Int J Pediatr Otorhinolaryngol 1992;23:141–149.
8 Kitsko DJ, Chi DH: Coblation removal of large suprastomal tracheal granulomas. Laryngoscope 2009;119:387–389.

Christopher J. Hartnick, MD
Professor, Department of Otology and Laryngology
Chief, Division of Pediatric Otolaryngology
Director, Pediatric Airway, Voice and Swallowing Center
Chief Quality Officer
Massachusetts Eye and Ear Infirmary, Harvard Medical School
243 Charles Street
Boston, MA 02116 (USA)
E-Mail christopher_hartnick@meei.harvard.edu

Hartnick CJ, Hansen MC, Gallagher TQ (eds): Pediatric Airway Surgery. Adv Otorhinolaryngol. Basel, Karger, 2012, vol 73, pp 66–69

Thyroglossal Duct Cyst Excision

Thomas Q. Gallagher[a] · Christopher J. Hartnick[b]

[a]LCDR, MC, USN, Department of Otolaryngology, Naval Medical Center Portsmouth, Portsmouth, Va., [b]Department of Otology and Laryngology, Massachusetts Eye & Ear Infirmary, Boston, Mass., USA

Abstract

Thyroglossal duct cysts (TGDCs) are the most common congenital anomaly of the neck. The most common presentation of TGDCs is a firm, midline mass. The Sistrunk procedure is the recommended treatment for TGDCs. Based on anatomic and embryologic study, Dr. Sistrunk recommended removal of not only the cyst and central portion of the hyoid bone, but also a central core of deep tongue musculature. By doing so, the rate of recurrence is decreased from approximately 50 to 3–5%. In this chapter, the authors will describe the Sistrunk procedure step by step including surgical pearls for success.

Thyroglossal duct cysts (TGDCs) are the most common congenital anomaly of the neck. They can form anywhere along the potential space formed by the path of the embryonic TGD from the foramen cecum to the orthotopic thyroid gland. They are frequently located in the perihyoid area (98%) and are rarely located intralingually, suprasternally,

or intrathyroidally [1]. The most common presentation of TGDCs is a firm midline mass. However, up to 20% of TGDCs can be off midline [2]. The patient may have a history of previous drainage or infection at the site or it may just present as a painless mass. It is classically described on physical exam as moving cephalad with tongue protrusion.

The Sistrunk procedure is the recommended treatment for TGDCs. Based on anatomic and embryologic study, Dr. Sistrunk recommended removal of not only the cyst and central portion of the hyoid bone, but also a central core of deep tongue musculature [3]. By doing so, the rate of recurrence is decreased from approximately 50 to 3–5%. [4].

Recurrence of TGDCs can be troublesome often requiring a central neck dissection in order to remove the recurrent cyst. Factors associated with TGDC recurrence range from inaccurate initial diagnosis, to infection, unusual TGDC presentation, and lack of BOT musculature removal [5].

Relevant Anatomy

Maddalozzo et al. [1] in 2010 described the posterior hyoid space as it relates to the excision of TGDCs. Histologic and cadaveric dissection

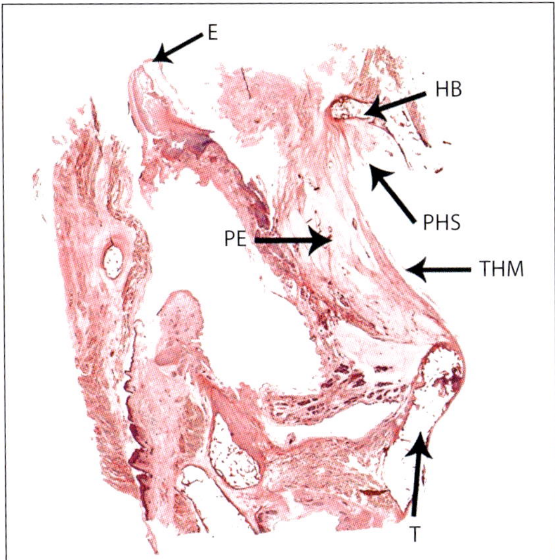

Fig. 1. Whole-mount human larynx prepared in the sagittal plane illustrating the anatomy described. Note: The thyrohyoid membrane (THM) does not insert on the inferior rim of the hyoid. E = Epiglottis; HB = hyoid bone; PE = preepiglottic space; PHS = posterior hyoid space; T = thyroid cartilage. Reprinted with kind permission from [1].

demonstrates that the thyrohyoid membrane inserts on the superior rim of the hyoid bone (fig. 1, 2). It is important for surgeons to conceptualize this relationship when removing TGDCs.

Indications

- Surgical excision is recommended for TGDCs since they have a propensity for recurrent infection and a very low risk of malignancy
- Active infections should be treated with antibiotics and/or drainage prior to formal excision in order to reduce surgical complications and decrease chances of recurrence

Contraindications

None.

Anesthesia Considerations

The endotracheal tube should be taped to the upper lip to facilitate access to the mouth in case palpation of the base of tongue becomes necessary during the procedure

Preparation

- An ultrasound of the neck mass is usually performed during the workup of the pediatric midline neck mass. It is important to confirm a normal, orthotopic thyroid gland. Lack of one will not change the decision for surgical management but will assist with postoperative management and surgical consent.
- If no normal orthotopic thyroid is present, thyroid function testing should be performed as well as a referral to endocrinology
- A generous shoulder roll is used to expose the neck mass

Procedure

- A transverse, midline cervical skin incision is marked out just inferior to the neck mass and injected with local anesthetic (fig. 3)
- If the neck mass has overlying skin changes, it may be excised with the skin incision
- An incision is carried down through the platysma layer (online suppl. video 1). Care is taken to avoid violating the cyst. 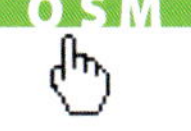
- If the cyst is violated, ensure complete dissection around the cyst wall in order to remove all components of the cyst
- Skin flaps are elevated superiorly to the level of the hyoid bone and inferiorly to identify the cricothyroid region
- Dissection deep to the inferior margin of the cyst is performed, dividing the strap muscles in the midline

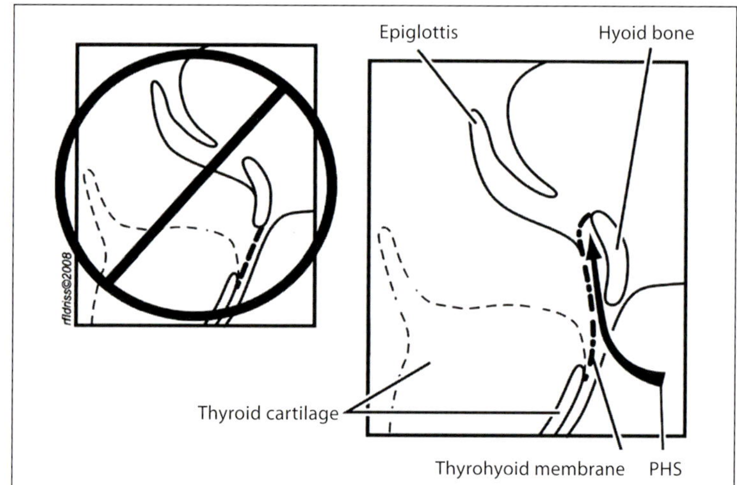

Fig. 2. A drawing of the base of tongue and upper laryngeal area. The dotted line demonstrates the thyrohyoid membrane's primary insertion on the preepiglottic tissues and its reflection and the attachment on the superior rim of the hyoid. Arrow indicates PHS. Reprinted with kind permission from [1].

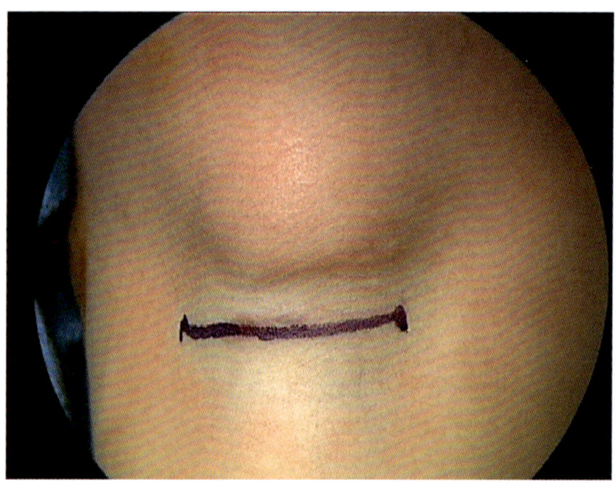

Fig. 3. A transverse, midline cervical skin incision is marked out just inferior to the neck mass and injected with local anesthetic.

- The trachea and thyroid are identified as well as the thyroid cartilage and thyroid notch
- The cyst and posterior hyoid space contents are then dissected off the thyroid cartilage up to the level of the hyoid bone
- This differs from recurrent and revision TGDC excisions where a more aggressive central neck dissection is performed to ensure removal of any cyst or tract remnant

- The hyoid bone is grasped with an Allis clamp to facilitate dissection
- The suprahyoid/infrahyoid musculature is dissected off the paramedian portion of the hyoid bone (medial to the central tendon of the digastric muscle) to allow easy division of the bone with Mayo scissors
- If the tract of the duct continues superiorly, it is dissected free along with a cuff of tongue musculature
- If necessary, a gloved finger placed in the mouth can assist the surgeon in determining the depth of dissection into the tongue musculature and to prevent violation of the oropharynx
- Once the cyst is removed, the wound is copiously irrigated with sterile saline and hemostasis is achieved with cautery where necessary (fig. 4)
- The strap muscles are reapproximated over a passive drain using 3-0 absorbable, braided suture in a running fashion
- The skin is closed in a layered fashion with absorbable suture and a thyroid compression dressing is placed

Gallagher · Hartnick

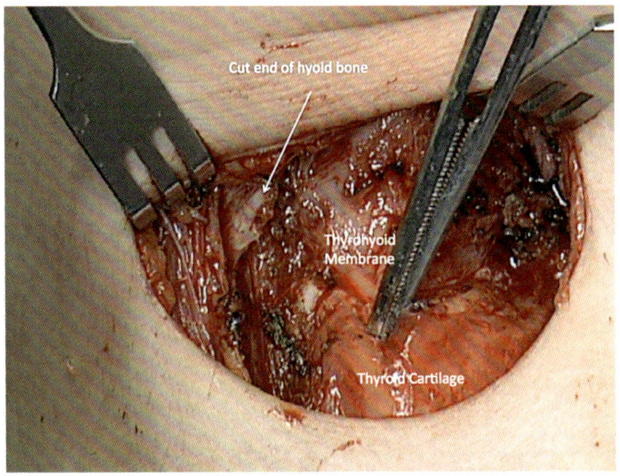

Fig. 4. The surgical field after resection of the TGD, hyoid bone and posterior hyoid space contents. The thyroid notch is demonstrated with a hemostat for orientation.

Postoperative Care

- The patient is observed overnight to evaluate for hematoma or any airway compromise, and the drain is removed the following day
- Antibiotics other than standard perioperative antibiotics are seldom necessary unless there are concerns for active infection

Pearls

- Actively infected TGDCs are allowed to 'cool off' with a course of antibiotics and needle aspiration, if necessary, prior to performing a more definitive excision
- Identification of the thyroid notch and thyroid cartilage are essential to ensure the proper plane of dissection during cyst removal
- If there have been previous infections of the cyst, the medial portions of the strap muscles may be adherent to the cyst making the plane of dissection difficult to find. A medial portion of strap muscle may be included with the specimen in these cases.
- Utilizing the Allis clamp for counter-traction during dissection of the hyoid bone is extremely helpful
- If a pharyngotomy is created during removal of the deep tongue musculature, it is closed in several layers
- Recurrent TGDCs are treated more aggressively, a central neck dissection is carried out where the entire central neck contents, between the strap muscles, are removed and the deep plane is carried down to the laryngotracheal framework

References

1 Maddalozzo J, Alderfer J, Mondi V: Posterior hyoid space as related to excision of the thyroglossal duct cyst. Laryngoscope 2010;120:1773–1778.
2 Walton BR, Koch KE: Presentation in management of a thyroglossal duct cyst with papillary carcinoma. South Med J 1997;90:758–761.

3 Sistrunk WE: Technique of removal of cysts and sinuses of the thyroglossal duct. Surg Gynecol Obstet 1928;46:109 –112.
4 Brown PM, Judd ES: Thyroglossal duct cysts and sinuses: results of radical Sistrunk operation. Am J Surg 1961;102:494–501.

5 Perkins JA, Inglis AF, Sie KC, Manning SC: Recurrent thyroglossal duct cysts: a 23-year experience and a new method for management. Ann Otol Rhinol Laryngol 2006;115:850–856.

Christopher J. Hartnick, MD
Professor, Department of Otology and Laryngology
Chief, Division of Pediatric Otolaryngology
Director, Pediatric Airway, Voice and Swallowing Center
Chief Quality Officer,
Massachusetts Eye and Ear Infirmary, Harvard Medical School
243 Charles Street
Boston, MA 02116 (USA)
E-Mail christopher_hartnick@meei.harvard.edu

Hartnick CJ, Hansen MC, Gallagher TQ (eds): Pediatric Airway Surgery. Adv Otorhinolaryngol. Basel, Karger, 2012, vol 73, pp 70–75

Bilateral Submandibular Gland Excision and Parotid Duct Ligation

Thomas Q. Gallagher[a] · Christopher J. Hartnick[b]

[a]LCDR, MC, USN, Department of Otolaryngology, Naval Medical Center Portsmouth, Portsmouth, Va., [b]Department of Otology and Laryngology, Massachusetts Eye & Ear Infirmary, Boston, Mass., USA

Abstract

Sialorrhea affects a significant number of children with cerebral palsy and other neuromuscular disorders. It can lead not only to social embarrassment but also to severe medical issues including chronic aspiration. There are numerous medical and surgical options, which include oral medications and transdermal patches, botulinum injection, and various forms of surgical ligation or excision of the major salivary glands. In this chapter, the authors describe the surgical management of sialorrhea, highlighting surgical pearls necessary for success.

Sialorrhea or drooling is defined as the inability to control oral secretions. It can cause significant social and medical issues in children with neuromuscular disorders, the most common being cerebral palsy [1]. Anywhere from 10 to 58% of children with cerebral palsy suffer from chronic sialorrhea [2]. Sialorrhea differs from ptyalism in that it is

The views expressed in this article are those of the authors and do not necessarily reflect the official policy or position of the Department of the Navy, Department of Defense, or the United States Government.

Thomas Q. Gallagher is a military service member. This work was prepared as part of his official duties. Title 17 .S.C. 105 provides that 'Copyright protection under this title is not available for any work of the United States Government.' Title 17 U.S.C. 101 defines a United States Government work as a work prepared by a military service member or employee of the United States Government as part of that person's official duties.

not due to excessive saliva production, rather the inability to properly manage saliva secondary to impaired oropharyngeal muscle control. The majority (70%) of saliva is produced by the submandibular, sublingual, and parotid glands [3]. Of these glands, the submandibular and sublingual produce about 2/3 of the basal salivary flow. The parotid gland produces saliva during meals.

Medical options to control chronic sialorrhea include behavior modification and biofeedback, medications such as anticholinergics, and injection of botulism toxin into the salivary glands under ultrasound guidance. Anticholinergic medications in particular are not always effective and have side effects, which can include urinary retention and constipation.

Surgical options to treat sialorrhea resulting in chronic aspiration are laryngotracheal separation, tracheotomy, bilateral submandibular gland excision and parotid duct ligation (BSGE-PDL), four-duct ligation (bilateral submandibular and parotid gland ducts) and chorda tympani nerve section. The first two are not usually considered first-line surgical treatment for chronic sialorrhea and are indicated when there is significant, recurrent aspiration. Neurectomy has not been found to be effective, risks damage to the hearing mechanism and leads to loss of taste [4]. Four-

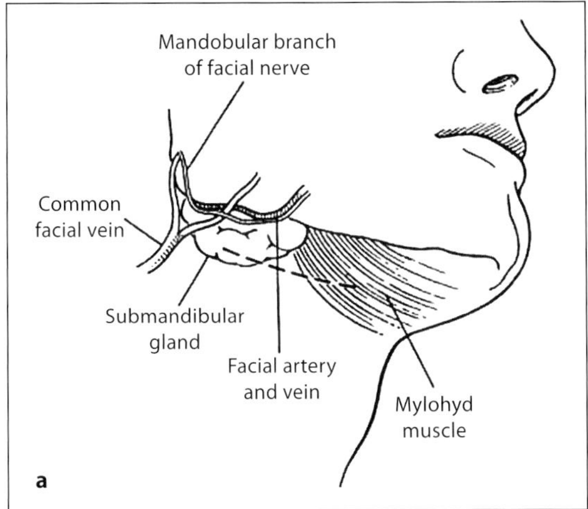

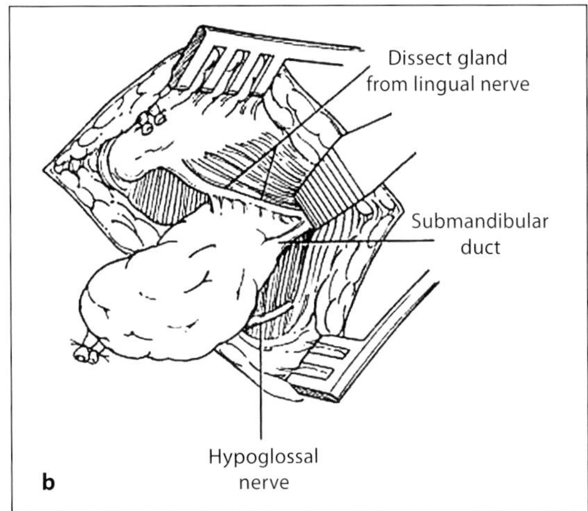

Fig. 1. a Incision used to perform submandibular gland resection (dotted line) with important anatomic structures shown. **b** Mylohyoid muscle is retracted to expose the submandibular duct and lingual nerve. Reprinted with kind permission from Khatri V, Operative Surgery Manual, 2003, Elsevier.

duct ligation and BSGE-PDL have been shown to have the best success rates (81 and 86–88%, respectively) [5–8].

There has been debate in the literature regarding decreased salivary flow rates being cariogenic. In a recent randomized controlled trial looking at botulism toxin injected into parotid and submandibular glands, Wu et al. [9] found that the decreased salivary flow rate has a negligible influence on salivary pH level and cariogenic bacterial amount.

Relevant Anatomy

- The submandibular gland is located within the submandibular triangle. This triangle is bounded by the mandible superiorly and the anterior and posterior bellies of the digastric muscle (fig. 1).
- Relevant neurovascular structures
- Marginal mandibular branch of the facial nerve (CN VII)
- Hypoglossal nerve (CN XII)
- Lingual nerve (CN V)

- The parotid duct is usually identifiable by its associated papilla. This can be found on the buccal mucosa adjacent to the 2nd maxillary molar.

Indications

- Parents of children with sialorrhea are initially offered botulin toxin injection into the parotid and submandibular glands to gauge improvement in symptoms and quality of life. If they are pleased and do not want to have repetitive procedures requiring an anesthetic, they are offered BSGE-PDL.
- Chronic sialorrhea causing significant social isolation due to unpleasant odor or hygiene problems, embarrassment, discomfort, complicating patient care including irritated facial skin, increased oral and perioral infections, and dehydration [3]
- Children with neurologic or muscle conditions suffering from chronic sialorrhea
- Chronic aspiration of saliva

– If significant, discussion with the parents regarding placement of a tracheotomy to improve pulmonary toilet. The authors reserve laryngotracheal separation as the last and final intervention.

Contraindications

Reversible neurologic condition for which the sialorrhea is not considered permanent.

Anesthesia Considerations

- Nasotracheal intubation is preferred but not required in order to have wide access to the oral cavity
- Location of the anesthesia machine so that there is access to the head of the bed as well as both sides of the patient; ideally the machine should be placed towards the patient's feet

Preparation

- Shoulder roll for exposure of the neck
- The patient should be prepped and draped to perform the submandibular gland excision first (see online suppl. video 1) followed by the PDL (see online suppl. video 2) in order to maintain sterility

Procedures

Submandibular Gland Excision
- Two 2- to 3-cm incisions are marked out approximately 1–2 fingerbreadths (~2 cm) below the inferior edge of the mandible in the orientation of the relaxed skin tension lines on either side of the neck (fig. 2)
- The incision is injected with 1% lidocaine with 1:100,000 epinephrine

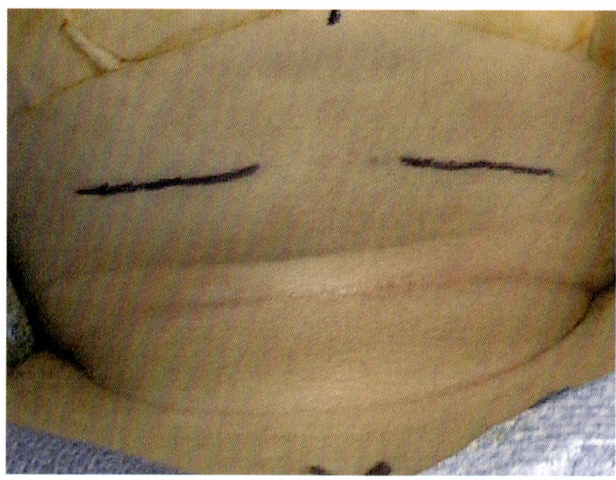

Fig. 2. Preoperative markings.

- Incision down through the platysma muscle with a scalpel
- Using a fine hemostat and bipolar cautery, dissection continues through the superficial layer of the deep cervical fascia
- Care is taken to keep the dissection towards the inferior portion of the wound to keep clear of the marginal mandibular nerve
- The submandibular gland is intermittently palpated through the wound during the dissection in order to determine its location and expose its inferior surface
- The common facial vein is usually encountered during this part of the dissection
- Dividing the common facial vein and reflecting it superiorly (Hayes-Martin maneuver) will protect the marginal mandibular branch of the facial nerve
- Once the inferior surface of the gland has been exposed, a Babcock clamp is placed on the inferior gland to assist with traction and countertraction
- Dissection continues superiorly along the capsule of the gland both on the superficial and deep surfaces
- The digastric muscle and the hypoglossal nerve are identified and preserved deep to the submandibular gland (fig. 3)

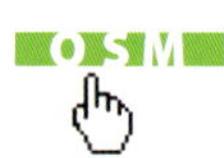

Gallagher · Hartnick

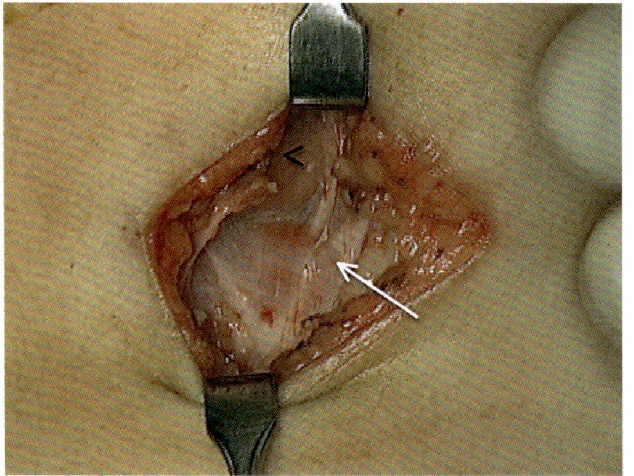 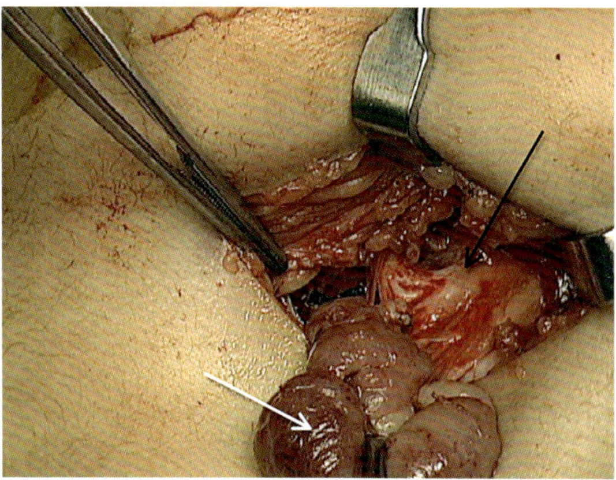

Fig. 3. The exposure of the inferior submandibular gland (SMG) on the right. The black arrowhead is the SMG and the white arrow is the anterior belly of the digastric muscle.

Fig. 4. The white arrow points to the right SMG retracted inferiorly using the Babcock clamp, the black arrow demonstrates the lingual nerve. Anteriorly (right), a Senn retractor is reflecting the mylohyoid muscle to help expose the lingual nerve and Wharton's duct.

- Dissection on the gland posteriorly will expose the anterior sternocleidomastoid muscle as well as the facial artery
- In some cases, the artery can be dissected free of the gland by dividing the small contributions to the gland
- In other cases the artery is intimately associated with the gland necessitating its division (possibly twice)
- Anteriorly, the dissection involves removing the superficial portion of the gland off the mylohyoid muscle
- During this part of the dissection, the use of bipolar is recommended as there are numerous small vessels between the gland and the mylohyoid muscle
- The posterior edge of the mylohyoid is retracted anteriorly with either a Senn retractor or Army-Navy retractor
- This helps expose the deep portion of the submandibular gland as well as its attachment to the submandibular ganglion and lingual nerve (fig. 4)
- The gland attachments to the submandibular ganglion are divided with bipolar cautery

- The last remaining attachment is anterior and consists of the submandibular duct or Wharton's duct
- This is clamped, divided and tied off with silk suture
- The wound bed (fig. 5) is then examined and irrigated; a Valsalva maneuver to 30 cm H_2O pressure is performed to check for hemostasis
- The wound is closed in layers using absorbable suture over a passive drain (fig. 6)
- Care is taken when reapproximating the platysma muscle layer. One should not take a large 'bite' with the suture thus entrapping the marginal mandibular nerve.

Parotid Duct Ligation
- Exposure of the parotid duct is facilitated with use of any of the following
- Small bite block
- Medesy mouth gag (aka 'side-biter')
- Wieder tongue retractor (aka 'sweetheart')
- Minnesota retractor
- Army-Navy retractor
- Once the punctum is identified, a Bowman lacrimal probe is used to cannulate the duct

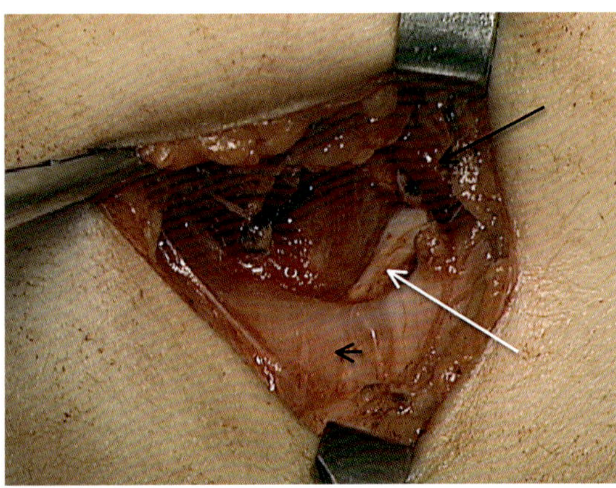

Fig. 5. The wound bed after the right SMG is removed with exposure of the digastric muscle (black arrowhead), hypoglossal nerve (white arrow), and the posterior edge of the mylohyoid muscle (black arrow). A silk tie is seen on the stump of the facial artery.

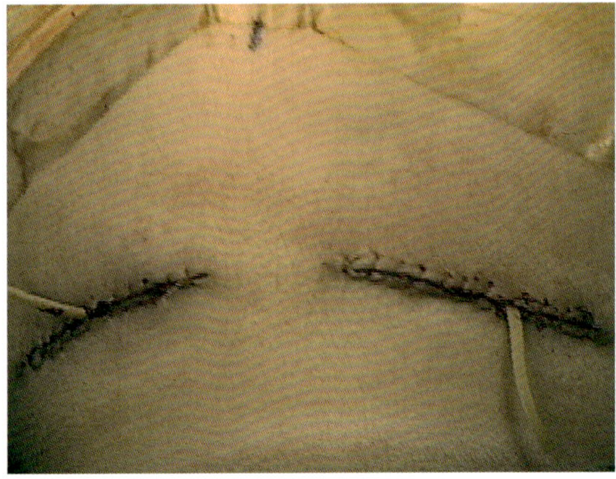

Fig. 6. The postoperative view with passive drains in place.

- Drying the buccal mucosa with a sponge, massaging the ipsilateral gland, and observing salivary flow will assist with punctum location
- Loupe magnification is helpful in identifying the punctum
- Bovie electrocautery with a Colorado tip (setting of 10 W on coagulation) is used to create an ellipse around the punctum

- An Allis clamp is used to grasp both the punctum and lacrimal probe to provide traction
- The duct is then dissected free of the enveloping buccinator muscle using the electrocautery
- Enough of the duct is dissected free in order to adequately suture ligate the duct, usually this is about 1 cm
- A suture ligature is then performed using 2-0 silk on a tapered needle
- The mucosa around the punctum is removed and the ligated duct is buried by closing the buccal mucosa using 4-0 chromic sutures

Postoperative Care

- Perioperative antibiotics are recommended
- The passive drains are usually removed on postoperative day one, but may be left in longer if there is significant drainage
- Patients can experience painful swelling of the parotid glands for several weeks after this procedure. The authors recommend use of appropriate pain medication as well as a 6-week course of an anti-staphylococcal antibiotic to prevent sialadenitis.

Pearls

- Utilizing the Hayes-Martin maneuver to preserve the marginal mandibular nerve
- Bipolar electrocautery when dissecting the superior portion of the submandibular gland off the mylohyoid muscle
- Retracting the posterior edge of the mylohyoid muscle anteriorly in order to identify the lingual nerve adequately
- Loupe magnification during location and cannulation of the parotid duct punctum

References

1 Harris S, Purdy A: Drooling and its management in cerebral palsy. Dev Med Child Neurol 1987;29:805–814.
2 Tahmassebi JF, Curzon ME, Curzon MEJ: Prevalence of drooling in children with cerebral palsy attending special schools. Dev Med Child Neurol 2003;45:613–617.
3 Cotton RT, Richardson MA: The effect of submandibular duct rerouting in the treatment of sialorrhea in children. Otolaryngol Head Neck Surg 1981;89:535–541.
4 Michel RG, Johnson KA, Patterson CN: Parasympathetic nerve section for control of sialorrhea. Arch Otolaryngol 1977;103:94–97.
5 Shirley WP, Hill JS, Woolley AL, Wiatrak BJ: Success and complications of four-duct ligation for sialorrhea. Int J Ped Otolaryngol 2003;67:1–6.
6 Shott SR, Myer CM, Cotton RT: Surgical management of sialorrhea. Otolaryngol Head Neck Surg 1989;101:47–50.
7 Dundas DF, Peterson RA: Surgical treatment of drooling by bilateral parotid duct ligation and submandibular gland resection. Plast Reconstr Surg 1979;64:47–51.
8 Brundage SR, Moore WD: Submandibular gland resection and bilateral parotid duct ligation as a management for chronic drooling in cerebral palsy. Plast Reconstr Surg 1989;83:443–446.
9 Katie Pei-Hsuan Wu, Jyh-Yuh Ke, Chung-Yao Chen, et al: A randomized, double-blind, placebo-controlled study botulinum toxin type A on oral health in treating sialorrhea in children with cerebral palsy. J Child Neurol 2011;26:838–843.

Thomas Q. Gallagher
LCDR, MC, USN
Naval Medical Center Portsmouth
Department of Otolaryngology, Bldg 3, 4th Floor
620 John Paul Jones Circle
Portsmouth, VA 23708 (USA)
E-Mail thomasqgallagher@yahoo.com

Hartnick CJ, Hansen MC, Gallagher TQ (eds): Pediatric Airway Surgery. Adv Otorhinolaryngol. Basel, Karger, 2012, vol 73, pp 76–79

Tracheocutaneous Fistula Closure

Thomas Q. Gallagher[a] · Christopher J. Hartnick[b]

[a]LCDR, MC, USN, Department of Otolaryngology, Naval Medical Center Portsmouth, Portsmouth, Va., [b]Department of Otology and Laryngology, Massachusetts Eye & Ear Infirmary, Boston, Mass., USA

Abstract

Tracheocutaneous fistula (TCF) is one of the recognized sequelae of tracheotomy in the pediatric age group. Persistent TCF can cause considerable morbidity due to recurrent aspiration, and subsequent respiratory infection, difficulty in phonation, ineffective cough, skin irritation, cosmesis, social acceptance, and intolerance to submersion. Methods of TCF closure remain controversial and vary based on the otolaryngologist's preference. The authors' choice is fistulectomy with primary closure in layers as this definitively removes the fistula and provides the patient with a good cosmetic result without the need for any significant postoperative wound care. The following chapter describes our techniques as well as surgical pearls for success.

Tracheocutaneous fistula (TCF) is one of the recognized sequelae of tracheotomy in the pediatric age group. Its incidence ranges widely from 3.3 to 43%, and persistence of TCF is related to duration of cannulation, age of tracheostomy, and technique employed [1, 2]. Tasca and Clarke [1]

recently published their 14-year experience with pediatric tracheostomy and reported an 11.9% rate of persistent TCF. Epithelialization and cicatricial scarring are thought to be responsible for persistence of the tract; however, maturation of the stoma with sutures at the time of surgery has not been shown to increase the incidence of fistula [3]. Kulber and Passy [4] reported that a fistula does not develop when cannulation is less than 16 weeks, but incidence increases to 70% when the cannulation period is greater than 16 weeks. Others have reported that the rate of TCF is 50% after cannulation for one year.

Persistent TCF can cause considerable morbidity due to recurrent aspiration, and subsequent respiratory infection, difficulty in phonation, ineffective cough, skin irritation, cosmesis, social acceptance, and intolerance to submersion.

Methods of TCF closure remain controversial and vary based on the otolaryngologist's preference. They include primary closure in layers, fistulectomy and primary closure in layers, and fistulectomy with healing by secondary intention as mentioned by Dr. Bluestone [2, 5–7]. Eaton et al. [8] from UT Southwestern describes using monopolar cauterization to close their TCFs. The authors' choice is fistulectomy with primary closure in layers, as this definitively removes the fistula and provides the patient with a good cosmetic result without the need for any significant postoperative wound care.

The time between decannulation and TCF closure varies in the literature as well. Reported time periods have been as short as 3 months and as long as 12 years; however, after a review of the literature most authors seem to pursue closure if the fistula has been present for at least 3–6 months or if there were pressing clinical concerns (i.e. persistent skin irritation or breakdown, difficulty with phonation) [7, 9]. The time period of 3–6 months between decannulation and TCF closure otherwise seems arbitrary perhaps based on the reasonably expected time for a stoma to granulate closed.

Indications

- Recurrent aspiration and subsequent respiratory infection
- Difficulty in phonation
- Ineffective cough
- Skin irritation
- Cosmesis and social acceptance
- Intolerance to submersion

Contraindications

- Chronic cough or recent upper respiratory infection
- Moderate to severe tracheomalacia
- Ventilator dependence
- Need for continued pulmonary toilet
- Decannulated in the previous 3–6 months
- Inability to expose the child's larynx to the point where the airway would be deemed 'unsafe' (Pierre Robin Sequence, severe trismus, etc.)
- Relative indication: failed polysomnogram (with stoma occluded)

Anesthesia Considerations

There is a risk of airway fire due to the use of electrocautery near the trachea. A discussion with the anesthesiologist is necessary regarding decreasing the oxygen percentage during that time.

Preparation

- Preoperative polysomnogram if concerns for obstructive sleep symptoms
- Perform with occlusive dressing over fistula
- It is important to perform direct laryngoscopy and bronchoscopy prior to TCF closure
- Rule out causes of possible airway obstruction such as peristomal granulation tissue
- Determine if the patient would have a difficult intubation and removal of the tracheostomy tube would pose a safety concern
- Failure to do so may lead to unexpected respiratory arrest, reintubation or recannulation
- A shoulder roll is necessary to expose the neck appropriately

Procedure

- The patient is prepped and draped in a sterile fashion for an anterior neck case
- An ellipse is marked out incorporating the fistula tract and injected with 1% lidocaine with 1:100,000 epinephrine (online suppl. video 1)
- An incision through the skin and subcutaneous tissues is performed with a scalpel
- The tissues surrounding the fistula tract tend to have significant scar from inflammation and tend to be thick
- Blunt dissection along the fistula tract is performed down to the level of the trachea
- The scar may be difficult to dissect and a curved iris scissor may be helpful
- Bipolar cautery is used for hemostasis
- Care is taken to avoid violating the fistula tract during the dissection
- The fistula tract is followed as it enters the trachea then sharply divided

- The trachea is then closed with simple interrupted sutures using 4-0 absorbable braided suture
- Fibrin tissue sealant is then placed over the trachea prior to closure of the strap muscles
- The strap muscles are reapproximated with a running 4-0 braided, absorbable suture over a passive drain
- The wound bed is then filled with sterile saline and a Valsalva maneuver to 30 cm H_2O pressure is performed to ensure the trachea is air tight (leak test)
- The subcutaneous tissues and skin are closed in a layered fashion using absorbable suture

Postoperative Care

- The patient is extubated and brought to the PICU for observation overnight
- Postoperative care varies in the literature
- Some prefer waking the patients up immediately after closure while others prefer keeping them intubated 18–24 h after operation
- Dr. Cotton's group did a retrospective review of 104 TCF closures over a 7-year period and found no significant correlation between duration of postoperative intubation and the outcome [2]. Outcome was defined as early and late complications and closure of the TCF.
- Additionally, postoperative intubation for 24 h after TCF closure is more expensive and can lead to possible laryngeal injury and increased morbidity
- The patient is kept on a clear diet overnight and advanced as tolerated to his/her home diet on postoperative day one

Complications

- A major concern when performing TCF closure is the escape of air into the subcutaneous tissues surrounding the trachea, mediastinum, and pleural cavity leading to subcutaneous (cervicofacial) emphysema, pneumomediastinum, and pneumothorax
- Precautions taken to decrease this risk include 'leak testing' the wound prior to closure using saline, extubating the patients in the recovery room when they are fully awake to avoid paroxysmal coughing during recovery, overnight intubation to allow for closure of the defect (see discussion above), and insertion of a drain to allow a route of air/blood escape
- Do not use CPAP for respiratory distress as this can exacerbate air escape into the soft tissues of the neck and chest
- If the above occurs, reintubation with a cuffed endotracheal tube for several days is necessary to allow the trachea to seal and allow reabsorption of the air

Pearls

- Patient selection is paramount
- Patients with chronic cough or if their underlying disease process has not resolved should not have their TCF closed
- Patients who cannot be intubated due to anatomic obstruction or severe trismus are not good candidates for TCF closure. They pose a risk in the immediate postoperative setting in the case of acute respiratory distress or expanding subcutaneous emphysema.
- The Valsalva maneuver checking for an air-tight seal and placement of a drain are necessary to avoid postoperative subcutaneous emphysema
- Placement of a drain (active or passive) is essential to prevent subcutaneous air accumulation and hematoma formation
- PICU observation overnight
- Tracheotomy set at bedside in the case of hematoma of subcutaneous air expansion leading to airway compromise

– Age-appropriate laryngoscope and endotracheal tube at bedside

– Adequate discussion with the PICU team regarding possible overnight emergencies and points of contact in case of emergency

References

1 Tasca R, Clarke R: Tracheocutaneous fistula following paediatric tracheostomy – a 14-year experience at Alder Hey Children's Hospital. Int J Pediatr Otorhinolaryngol 2010;74:711–712.

2 Stern Y, Cosenza M, Walner D, Cotton R: Management of persistent tracheocutaneous fistula in the pediatric age group. Ann Otol Rhinol Laryngol 1999;108:880–883.

3 Colman KL, Mandell DL, Simons JP: Impact of stoma maturation on pediatric tracheostomy-related complications. Arch Otolaryngol Head Neck Surg 2010;136:471–474.

4 Kulber H, Passy V: Tracheotomy closure and scar revisions. Arch Otolaryngol 1972;96:2–26.

5 Bishop JB, Bostwick J, Nekoi F: Persistent tracheal stoma. Am J Surg 1980;140:709–710.

6 Bluestone CD, Rosenfeld RM: Surgical Atlas of Pediatric Otolaryngology. Hamilton, BC Decker, 2002, pp 593–596.

7 Schroeder J, Greene R, Holinger L: Primary closure of tracheocutaneous fistula in pediatric patients. J Pediatr Surg 2008;43:1786–1790.

8 Eaton D, Brown O, Parry D: Simple technique for tracheocutaneous fistula closure in the pediatric population. Ann Otol Rhinol Laryngol 2003;112:17–19.

9 Geyer M, Kubba H, Hartley B: Experiences of tracheocutaneous fistula closure in children: how we do it. Clin Otolaryngol 2008;33:367–369.

Christopher J. Hartnick, MD
Professor, Department of Otology and Laryngology
Chief, Division of Pediatric Otolaryngology
Director, Pediatric Airway, Voice and Swallowing Center
Chief Quality Officer
Massachusetts Eye and Ear Infirmary, Harvard Medical School
243 Charles Street
Boston, MA 02116 (USA)
E-Mail christopher_hartnick@meei.harvard.edu

Hartnick CJ, Hansen MC, Gallagher TQ (eds): Pediatric Airway Surgery. Adv Otorhinolaryngol. Basel, Karger, 2012, vol 73, pp 80–85

Pediatric Ansa Cervicalis to Recurrent Laryngeal Nerve Anastomosis

Marshall E. Smith

Division of Otolaryngology/Head and Neck Surgery, Primary Children's Medical Center, University of Utah School of Medicine, Salt Lake City, Utah, USA

Abstract

This chapter reviews laryngeal reinnervation with ansa cervicalis for treatment of unilateral vocal fold paralysis and glottal incompetence in children. The relevant anatomy is discussed; the indications and contraindications are detailed. This is followed by a stepwise description of the surgical details of this operation.

The ideal surgical treatment for unilateral vocal fold paralysis in children or adults has not been established. Options for management include injection, medialization, and reinnervation. The advantages and disadvantages of these techniques continue to be actively debated. Unfortunately, there are few direct comparisons in outcomes between these various techniques. However, a recent report of a randomized prospective, multi-center surgical trial in 24 adults with unilateral vocal fold paralysis of medialization laryngoplasty vs. laryngeal reinnervation found that for patients under 50 years old reinnervation yielded better results than thyroplasty [1]. The only patients in the trial who were rated by blinded listeners as having normal voice quality were in the reinnervation group. These results imply that younger patients, including children, have more capability to regenerate peripheral nerves after neurorrhaphy.

The otolaryngologist must base treatment decisions on experience and judgment of the advantages and disadvantages of the different procedures. The decision regarding the preferred surgical approach is especially challenging in children in whom treatment effects should be long lasting, affording the child an optimal voice quality throughout their adult life. A lifelong voice disorder can affect their self-image, self-confidence, career opportunities, and social interactions.

Laryngeal reinnervation procedures have advantages in treatment of dysphonia from glottic incompetence due to unilateral vocal fold paralysis in the pediatric and adolescent age group. The procedure requires no foreign body implant that may extrude or migrate later in life. There is no injection material to resorb, shrink, or create an inflammatory granulomatous mass. Injection laryngoplasty is not a reasonable long-term treatment for children, because no long-term injectable implant is currently available; Radiesse® (calcium hydroxyapatite microspheres) which is currently

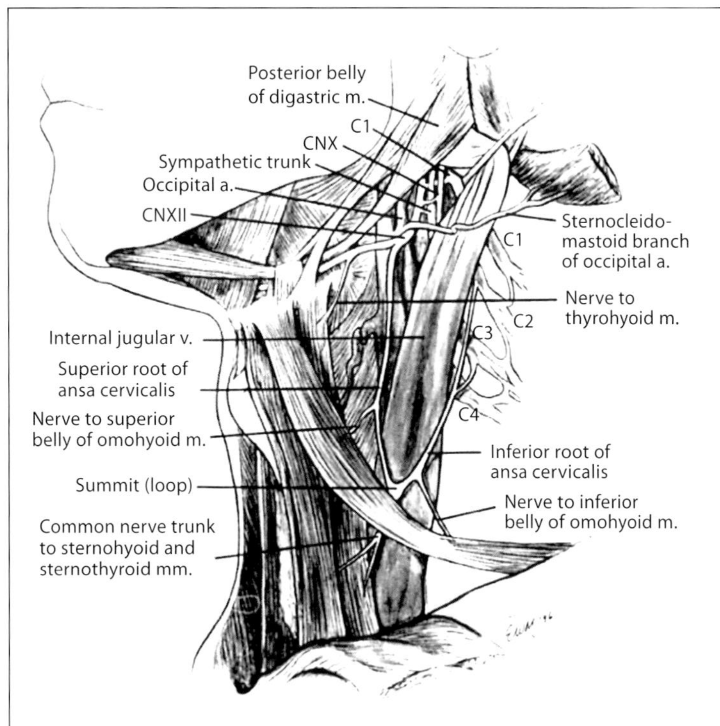

Fig. 1. Regional anatomy of the ansa cervicalis nerve. Reproduced from Chhetri and Berke [2] with permission.

in use undergoes gradual resorption. Its average benefit is 18 months, which is clearly not long enough for a child. The long-term side effects of the implant are also unknown. Additionally, local anesthesia needed for medialization laryngoplastic phonosurgery is not a realistic option for children or many adolescents. The reinnervation operation is done under general anesthesia, so that the fine adjustments required for medialization laryngoplasty under local anesthesia are not needed. Reinnervation is expected to maintain the vocal improvement throughout the patient's life. Laryngeal reinnervation may yield improved pitch and loudness control of the voice, as opposed to a static implant. The chief drawback of laryngeal reinnervation is the delay in time until the reinnervation increases laryngeal muscle tone sufficient to improve the voice. This usually takes 3–6 months, with an average of 4.5 months. This

disadvantage can be mitigated by performing vocal fold injection with a temporary filler material (e.g. Cymetra®) to provide improvement until the neurorrhaphy heals.

Relevant Anatomy

The ansa (Latin for 'handle of a cup') cervicalis nerve is a motor nerve from the C_2 and C_3 ventral rami that forms a loop with branches that innervate the strap muscles of the neck (fig. 1) [2]. These muscles include the omohyoid, sternohyoid, and sternothyroid muscles. The branch to the thyrohyoid muscle travels with the hypoglossal nerve before its entry into the muscle. The loop connects as the nerve crosses over the internal jugular vein. The nerve branches come off the loop and insert into the belly of the various strap

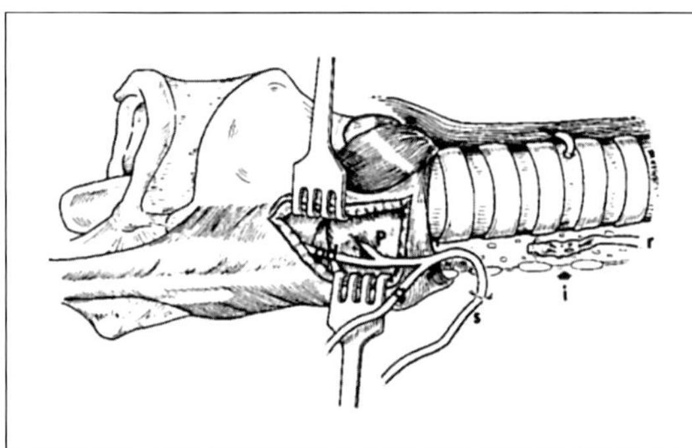

Fig. 2. Ansa cervicalis RLN anastomosis. The ansa branch is severely damaged distally and sutured to distal stump of the RLN. Figure shows ipsilateral anastomosis, but contralateral ansa can be easily transferred across midline for suture to the opposite RLN. i = Injury site of RLN; g = Galen's anastomosis; P = PCA and abductor branch; ad = adductor branch of RLN. Reproduced from Crumley et al. [3] with permission.

muscles. Anatomical variations of the ansa cervicalis are common; however, this generally does not preclude dissection of a branch of approximate size of and adequate length to the recurrent laryngeal nerve (RLN).

The RLN runs up from the chest and toward the larynx, coursing under the lobes of the thyroid gland. After reflection of the thyroid lobe medially, the RLN can be seen entering the larynx posterior to the cricothyroid joint. Occasionally, the nerve may bifurcate before entry into the larynx. An accessory communication with the sensory branch of the larynx, called Galen's anastomosis may also be found. The main trunk of the nerve, proximal to these branches, is generally used in the repair. However, if the RLN is damaged at this level from prior surgical trauma, the nerve can reliably be found by rotating the larynx medially and dissecting at its entry behind the cricothyroid joint and under the thyroid ala. Here, it will separate into adductor and abductor branches. A depiction of the RLN anastomosis to the ansa cervicalis branch is seen in figure 2.

Indications

It is beyond the scope of this chapter to summarize the causes of vocal fold paralysis in children, or provide details of evaluation of children with suspected vocal fold paralysis. In evaluating patients who are potential candidates for treatment, it is assumed that the cause has been identified, and the patient has been followed for sufficient time (usually at least 1 year) to allow for recovery on their own. Laryngeal nerves have a high capacity to at least partially reinnervate after injury, yielding sufficient improvement in glottal closure to improve voice and swallow without recovery of vocal fold mobility. In the pediatric age group, patients who have undergone a cardiac procedure (such as patent ductus arteriosus, PDA) ligation, coarctation of the aorta repair, heart transplant, tetralogy of Fallot repair, etc.) resulting in injury to the left RLN are the most common group who have unilateral vocal fold paralysis and may be candidates for treatment of dysphonia.

The severity of dysphonia in children, especially young children, can be difficult to assess. Parents often underestimate the severity of their child's voice problem. When the child is young, he/she may not consider the difficulty the child with a soft weak voice will have being heard outside the home. As the child begins schooling, his/her social world grows with increased vocal demands. In fact, parents may be prompted by extended family members or others to seek attention for their child's voice problem.

Assessment of the child's voice problem can be challenging for the clinician because of difficulty eliciting a representative phonation sample during conversation with a young child in a medical setting. Speech development may be delayed. Time is required to elicit the child's confidence to get them to talk. A speech-language pathologist experienced in pediatric voice is an invaluable asset in evaluating these patients.

- Unilateral vocal fold paralysis with dysphonia
- Dysphagia may or may not be present, especially with liquids
- Laryngoscopy or laryngostroboscopy that documents an immobile vocal fold with a glottal gap, yielding a weak breathy, soft voice

Contraindications

- Immobility of the cricoarytenoid joint
- Atrophy of the paralyzed vocal fold
- Bilateral vocal fold paralysis
- Paralysis for less than one year

Anesthesia Considerations

- The patient is intubated with an appropriate-sized endotracheal tube
- During the dissection and localization of the ansa cervicalis nerve, a portable nerve stimulator is used to confirm the nerve location and branches
- No neuromuscular blockade should be given during this dissection, and no lidocaine should be infiltrated into the soft tissue around the ansa cervicalis. These will interfere with stimulation and identification of the nerve.

Preparation

- Preoperative:
- Awake unsedated laryngoscopy to document vocal fold immobility
- Recording of voice and parent-surrogate or patient voice assessment
- Swallowing evaluation
- Intraoperative:
- Microlaryngoscopy after induction of general anesthesia, or at a prior endoscopy
- Palpate the cricoarytenoid joint and rule out arytenoid fixation

– Conduct laryngeal EMG to confirm the paralysis
– Prior to laryngeal reinnervation, vocal fold injection with a temporary filler substance (e.g. micronized acellular dermis – Cymetra) may be done to provide temporary improvement in voice while waiting for the neurorrhaphy to heal

Procedure

- After microlaryngoscopy, the patient is intubated with an appropriate endotracheal tube
- The neck is extended, and the appropriate side surgical site in the neck is prepped
- A skin incision is made in a skin fold crease at or just below the cricoid cartilage, extending laterally to the anterior border of the sternocleidomastoid muscle (online suppl. 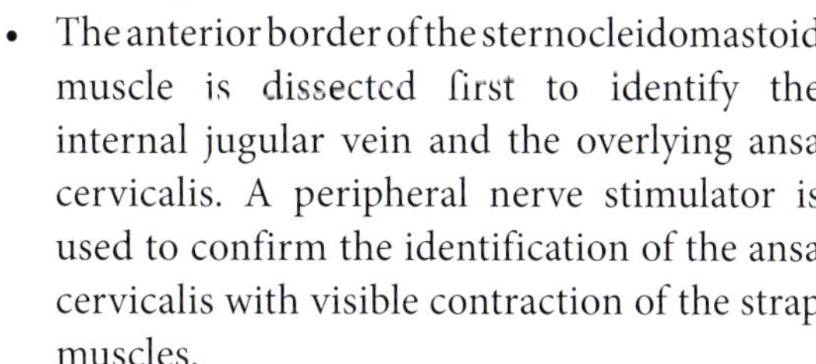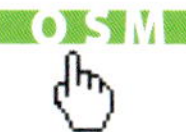 video 1)
- The anterior border of the sternocleidomastoid muscle is dissected first to identify the internal jugular vein and the overlying ansa cervicalis. A peripheral nerve stimulator is used to confirm the identification of the ansa cervicalis with visible contraction of the strap muscles.
- The nerve courses under the omohyoid muscle, so this muscle is dissected to facilitate mobilization of the nerve on either side of it
- The nerve is followed to the insertion of the branch to the sternohyoid and sternothyroid muscles low in the neck. The nerve is not transected yet.
- The thyroid lobe is dissected off the strap muscles and rotated medially to approach the tracheoesophageal groove. The superior or inferior pole vessels need not be ligated routinely, but the middle thyroid vein is ligated to rotate the lobe and expose the course of the RLN.

- If needed, to gain exposure to the cricothyroid joint where the RLN enters the larynx, the superior pole vessels may require ligation
- The RLN is identified and its course followed toward the larynx. Usually, a 1–1.5 cm length is dissected
  - If the nerve is damaged at its entry into the larynx (such as after thyroidectomy), the larynx is rotated medially to find the distal nerve stump
  - The ansa cervicalis nerve branch to the sternohyoid muscle is usually the longest available nerve to graft, and is an appropriate size match to the RLN
  - If not, the main trunk of the upper division of the ansa can be used, with transection of the loop across the internal jugular vein to provide enough length for the nerves to approximate without tension
  - A tunnel is created under the strap muscles, and the ansa cervicalis nerve is transposed to the RLN
  - An operating microscope is brought into the surgical field. Under magnification, the RLN is transected, and the distal RLN is sewn to the transposed ansa cervicalis with two or three 9-0 nylon sutures on a small spatula needle.
  - The wound is irrigated and closed in routine fashion
  - A passive surgical drain may or may not be used

Postoperative Care

- The patient is observed overnight and discharged the following day if the patient is without stridor, oral intake is adequate, and the surgical wound shows no sign of hematoma
- The wound is kept dry until a wound check 10–14 days postoperatively, at which time the bandage strips are removed if they have not come off

- The patient is seen at 4, 8, and 12 months postoperatively
- The final result of the procedure takes at least one year to assess. Patients usually begin to notice improvement in voice at 3–5 months, and the improvement continues for one year or more.

Pearls

- If the distal stump of the RLN is not found, then the ansa cervicalis can be implanted into the thyroarytenoid muscle by making a small window in the thyroid ala at the inferior border of the cartilage, opening the inner perichondrium, and implanting the nerve stump into the muscle through the paraglottic space. A nerve muscle pedicle of ansa cervicalis may also be used, but this author prefers direct nerve stump implantation. The voice results are comparable to direct neurorrhaphy [4].
- If the ansa cervicalis on the side of the paralysis is not found or has been injured from prior surgery, the other side of the neck can be explored to find an available ansa cervicalis donor nerve. The distal RLN is dissected with appropriate length to sew to the ansa branch from the other side. The anastomosis usually lies over the cricothyroid membrane [5].

Case Presentation

A 2-year-old male was born 30 weeks premature. He had a PDA that did not respond to medical treatment and underwent PDA ligation at 32 weeks of age. After extubation, he had a weak, soft cry and difficulty feeding. Flexible laryngoscopy identified left vocal fold paralysis. Aspiration was seen on a modified barium swallow, and a feeding tube was placed. These were continued until 4 months of life, when he was able to take thickened liquids. The patient was followed with flexible laryngoscopy at 6, 12, and 24 months of life. Left vocal fold paralysis was observed. Though his swallowing improved, he continued to cough with liquids. A soft voice persisted and his speech was delayed. His pediatric voice handicap index (pVHI) score was 15. The perceptual voice rating was G2R1B2A0S0. At 2 years of age, he underwent microlaryngoscopy and laryngeal EMG. This showed the left PCA had 2+ fibrillations and positive sharp waves, with a single motor unit firing at 20–30 Hz. The right PCA muscle had normal motor unit morphology and recruitment firing synchronously with inspiration. Given the length of time after injury, it was interpreted as unlikely to recover further. The patient was felt to be a good candidate for laryngeal reinnervation. Two months later, he underwent left ansa cervicalis to RLN reinnervation, and left vocal fold injection with Cymetra. His mother saw initial improvement in voice and swallowing after the procedure. This was attributed to the injection. Four months after the procedure his mother rated his voice at 85% normal, and he rarely choked with swallowing liquids. She reported that his cry and laugh were much louder, and his speech had also improved. pVHI score was 6, and perceptual voice rating was G1R1B0A0S0.

References

1 Paniello RC, Edgar JD, Kallogieri D, Piccarillo JC: Medialization vs. reinnervation for unilateral vocal fold paralysis: a multicenter randomized clinical trial. Laryngoscope 2011;121:1272–1279.
2 Chhetri D, Berke GS: Ansa cervicalis nerve: review of the topographic anatomy and morphology. Laryngoscope 1997;107:1366–1372.
3 Crumley RL, Izdebski K, McMicken B: Nerve transfer vs. Teflon injection for vocal cord paralysis; a comparison. Laryngoscope 1988;98:1200–1204.
4 Zheng H, Zhou S, Chen S, Li Z, Cuan Y: An experimental comparison of different kinds of laryngeal muscle reinnervation. Otolaryngol Head Neck Surg 1998;119:540–547.
5 Wang W, Chen S, Chen D, Xia S, Qiu X, Liu Y, Zheng H: Contralateral ansa cervicalis-to-recurrent laryngeal nerve anastomosis for unilateral vocal fold paralysis: a long-term outcome analysis of 56 cases. Laryngoscope 2011;121:1027–1034.

Marshall E. Smith
3C-120 SOM
50 N. Medical Drive
Salt Lake City, UT 84132 (USA)
E-Mail marshall.smith@hsc.utah.edu

Hartnick CJ, Hansen MC, Gallagher TQ (eds): Pediatric Airway Surgery. Adv Otorhinolaryngol. Basel, Karger, 2012, vol 73, pp 86–89

Pediatric Laryngeal Electromyography

Stephen C. Maturo[a] · Christopher J. Hartnick[b]

[a]Department of Otolaryngology, San Antonio Military Medical Center, Fort Sam Houston, Tex.,
[b]Department of Otology and Laryngology, Massachusetts Eye & Ear Infirmary, Boston, Mass., USA

Abstract

Vocal fold immobility (VFI) is a challenging management issue in pediatric otolaryngology. VFI is most commonly distinguished between unilateral (UVFI) and bilateral (BVFI) dysfunction. UVFI and BVFI are different pathophysiologic and clinical entities with distinct symptoms and etiologies. It has been generally accepted in the adult literature to wait at least 1 year prior to carrying out more permanent type procedures for VFI. This period has been extended out even further in children as the literature has suggested that vocal fold function may return many years later. Unfortunately, there is no simple test or procedure to help predict return of vocal fold function. In adult patients LEMG has been used to help guide management decisions, but it has not been widely investigated in children. In this chapter the authors describe a LEMG technique that has been a useful adjunct in managing children with VFI.

Vocal fold immobility (VFI) is a challenging management issue in pediatric otolaryngology.

Unilateral (UVFI) and bilateral (BVFI) VFI occur in equal incidences. UVFI is most commonly due to iatrogenic causes such as cardiothoracic surgery [1–6]. Congenital BVFI is the most common presentation of BVFI with various etiologies such as neurologic or idiopathic [1–6]. Management of UVFI and BVFI is also distinct with multiple interventions possible depending on the severity of the child's airway, voice, or swallowing symptoms. In children, it has been common practice to defer permanent laryngeal surgeries for years in anticipation that fold mobility will return. Unfortunately, there is no simple test or procedure to help predict return of vocal fold function. In adult patients, laryngeal electromyography (LEMG) has been used to help guide management decisions, but it has not been widely investigated in children [7–16].

The goal of this chapter is to describe the equipment and technique of pediatric LEMG. All equipment is readily available, and the technique for placement of the LEMG needles is a skill that pediatric endoscopists possess. The challenge is in the interpretation of the LEMG and using this information to help guide management. From this perspective, the reader should regard pediatric LEMG as one tool that may help physician, patients, and families make better, more informed decisions.

Indications

Children with UVFI or BVFI.

Contraindications

Children who cannot tolerate a general anesthetic.

Preoperative Preparation

- Flexible awake fiber-optic endoscopy is recommended to fully assess the movement of the vocal folds (see online suppl. video 1)
- In children with no apparent etiology for their VFI, imaging of the brain stem is recommended
- Clinical evidence of aspiration requires further investigation with a modified barium swallow study
- Surgical consent is similar to that of a direct laryngoscopy and bronchoscopy. Additional risks factors that may be mentioned include swelling of the vocal folds, vocal fold hematoma, and an inability to obtain accurate LEMG reading
- An experienced electromyographer is necessary to review the study. This technique allows for recording of the study so that the electromyographer does not need to be present during the procedure.
- Ensure that LEMG equipment is available and working prior to proceeding

Anesthesia Considerations

- An experienced anesthesiologist is recommended, especially one who is comfortable with maintaining spontaneous ventilation
- Communication between the surgeon and the anesthesiologist is critical to obtain the most accurate LEMG information

- Spontaneous ventilation is required. Avoid topical application of vocal folds as this may affect the results.
- One dose of intravenous steroids (usually dexamethasone 0.5 mg/kg up to 10 mg)
- Antibiotics are unnecessary

Equipment Needed

- See online supplementary PDF file 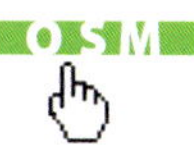
- Medtronic NIM Response 2.0: must have VGA and audio output
- Paired subdermal electrodes (Medtronic part number 8227410)
- Video converter 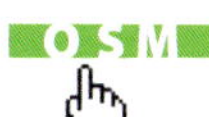
- Any unit that will convert VGA output to S-video or composite video will work
- The video converter converts the NIM output VGA to S-video allowing connection to digital video recorder. The author uses the following model: TView Micro (part No. 444-8600; Focus Enhancements Inc., Campbell, Calif., USA; http://www.focusinfo.com/solutions/catalog/asp?id = 151).
- Digital video recorder
- One can use any PC with video input card, video recording software, and CD/DVD burner
- Infant, pediatric, or adult Lindholm laryngoscope with suspension apparatus
- Laryngeal alligator forceps

Procedure

- See online supplementary PDF file, NIM settings pertaining to amplitude and sweep speed
- Place grounding leads
- After mask induction with general anesthetic, a total intravenous anesthesia technique is used
- The author's institution anesthesiologists usually use propofol and remifentanil

- The procedure begins with direct laryngoscopy and bronchoscopy for full airway evaluation
- Suspension laryngoscopy with an appropriate sized Lindholm laryngoscope
- Placement of laryngeal needle into thyroary-tenoid muscle
- If small larynx precludes both needles from recording simultaneously, then place the needles one side at a time (see online suppl. video 2)

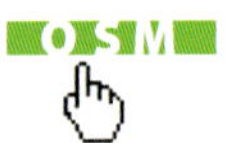

- Impedance values are confirmed; low impedance (<5) reflects accurate placement of electrodes, while high impedance required electrode repositioning
- Allow patient to emerge from anesthesia and begin recording
- If only able to test one side, then deepen patient and place needle in contralateral vocal fold
- Ensure that video has recorded

Postoperative Care

- Similar to that of a direct laryngoscopy
- Discharge on the same day of the procedure is reasonable
- The acoustic signal and video data are reviewed at a later time by an experienced electromyographer
- LEMGs are analyzed for the presence of normal-appearing motor unit action potentials (MUAPs), abnormal appearing MUAPs, and overall comparison between the two sides (see online suppl. videos 3 and 4)

Pearls

- The patient needs to be awakened or 'lightened up' from anesthetic in order to obtain accurate readings
- Given this, an experienced anesthesiologist is important
- When does one carry out an LEMG?
- Our experience with children with iatrogenic injuries would suggest that an optimal time period would be between 3 and 6 months after the injury [17]. Most likely, these children only require one LEMG.
- Children with congenital, idiopathic BVFI may need serial examinations prior to commenting on the likelihood of vocal fold return
- Interpreting LEMG must take the clinical scenario into context
- An LEMG in the setting of a child who underwent a PDA ligation and where there is no evidence of MUAP will unlikely regain vocal fold function
- A child with congenital, idiopathic VFI may have evidence of normal MUAPs on exam, but LEMG cannot definitively predict that this nerve will have full function or when function will return
- As with adult LEMG, future research is necessary to improve the technology and interpretation of pediatric LEMG

References

1 Daya H, Hosni A, Bejar-Solar I, Evans JN, et al: Pediatric vocal fold paralysis: a long term retrospective study. Arch Otolaryngol Head Neck Surg 2000;126:21–25.

2 Chen EY, Inglis AF: Bilateral vocal cord paralysis in children. Otolaryngol Clin North Am 2008;41:889–901.

3 Berkowitz RG: Natural history of tracheostomy-dependent idiopathic congenital vocal fold paralysis. Otolaryngol Head Neck Surg 2007;136:649–652.

4 Emery PJ, Fearon B: Vocal cord palsy in pediatric practice: a review of 71 cases. Int J Pediatr Otorhinolaryngol 1984;8:147–154.

5 Truong MT, Messner AH, Kerschner JE, Scholes M, et al: Pediatric vocal fold paralysis after cardiac surgery: rate of recovery and sequelae. Otolaryngol Head Neck Surg 2007;137:780–784.

6   Miyamoto CR, Parikh SR, Gellad W,
    Licameli GR: Bilateral congenital vocal
    cord paralysis. Otolaryngol Head Neck
    Surg 2005;133:241–245.
7   Berkowitz RG: Laryngeal electromyogra-
    phy findings in idiopathic congenital
    bilateral vocal cord paralysis. Ann Otol
    Rhinol Laryngol 1996;105:207–212.
8   Jacobs IN, Finkel RS: Laryngeal electro-
    myography in the management of vocal
    cord mobility problems in children. Lar-
    yngoscope 2002;112:1243–1248.
9   Wohl DL, Kilpatrick JK, Leshner RT,
    Shaia WT: Intraoperative pediatric
    laryngeal electromyography: experience
    and caveats with monopolar electrodes.
    Ann Otol Rhinol Laryngol 2001;110:
    524–531.
10 Koch BM, Milmoe G, Grundfast KM:
    Vocal cord paralysis in children studied
    by monopolar electromyography. Pediatr
    Neurol 1987;3:288–293.

11 Gartlan MG, Peterson KL, Hoffman HT,
    Luschei ES, et al: Bipolar hooked wire
    electromyographic technique in the eval-
    uation of pediatric vocal cord paralysis.
    Ann Otol Rhinol Laryngol 1993;102:
    695–700.
12 Berkowitz RG, Ryan MM, Pilowsky PM:
    Respiration-related laryngeal electro-
    myography in children with bilateral
    vocal fold paralysis. Ann Otol Rhinol
    Laryngol 2009;118:791–795.
13 Ysunza A, Landerso L, Pamplona C,
    Prado C, et al: The role of laryngeal elec-
    tromyography in the diagnosis of vocal
    fold immobility in children. Int J Pediatr
    Otorhinolaryngol 2007;71:949–958.
14 Scott AR, Siao Tick Chong P, Randolph
    G, Hartnick CJ: Intraoperative laryngeal
    electromyography in children with vocal
    fold immobility: a simplified technique.
    Int J Pediatr Otorhinolaryngol
    2008;72:31–40.

15 Scott AR, Siao Tick Chong P, Randolph
    G, Hartnick CJ: Spontaneous and evoked
    laryngeal electromyography of the thy-
    roarytenoid muscles: a canine model for
    intraoperative recurrent laryngeal nerve
    monitoring. Ann Otol Rhinol Laryngol
    2010;119:54–63.
16 Scott AR, Siao Tick Chong P, Brigger M,
    Randolph G, et al: Serial electroymyog-
    raphy of the thyroarytenoid muscles
    using the NIM-response system in a
    canine model of vocal fold paralysis.
    Ann Otol Rhinol Laryngol 2009;118:56–
    66.
17 Maturo SC, Braun N, Brown D, Kersch-
    ner J: Intraoperative laryngeal electro-
    myography (LEMG) in children with
    VFI: results of a multicenter longitudinal
    study. Arch Otolaryngol Head Neck
    Surg, in press.

Christopher J. Hartnick, MD
Professor, Department of Otology and Laryngology
Chief, Division of Pediatric Otolaryngology
Director, Pediatric Airway, Voice and Swallowing Center
Chief Quality Officer
Massachusetts Eye and Ear Infirmary, Harvard Medical School
243 Charles Street
Boston, MA 02116 (USA)
E-Mail christopher_hartnick@meei.harvard.edu

Hartnick CJ, Hansen MC, Gallagher TQ (eds): Pediatric Airway Surgery. Adv Otorhinolaryngol. Basel, Karger, 2012, vol 73, pp 90–94

Vocal Fold Injection Medialization Laryngoplasty

Vikash K. Modi

Pediatric Otolaryngology, Department of Otolaryngology- Head & Neck Surgery, Weill Cornell Medical College, New York, N.Y., USA

Abstract

Unilateral vocal fold paralysis (UVFP) can cause glottic insufficiency that can result in hoarseness, chronic cough, dysphagia, and/or aspiration. In rare circumstances, UVFP can cause airway obstruction necessitating a tracheostomy. The treatment options for UVFP include observation, speech therapy, vocal fold injection medialization laryngoplasty, thyroplasty, and laryngeal reinnervation. In this chapter, the author will discuss the technique of vocal fold injection for medialization of a UVFP.

Unilateral vocal fold paralysis (UVFP) can cause glottic insufficiency that can result in hoarseness, chronic cough, dysphagia, and/or aspiration. In rare circumstances, UVFP can cause airway obstruction necessitating a tracheostomy.

Etiologies of pediatric UVFP include birth trauma, central or peripheral neurologic anomalies, prolonged intubation, anoxia, cardiothoracic surgery, and idiopathic causes. Spontaneous recovery of congenital UVFP has been documented as late as 4 years of age in a child [1].

The treatment options for UVFP include observation, speech therapy, vocal fold injection medialization laryngoplasty, thyroplasty, and laryngeal reinnervation [2].

Materials utilized for vocal fold injection medialization laryngoplasty are autologous fat, gelatin sponge (Gelfoam; Pfizer, New York, New York), hydrated porcine gelatin powder (Surgifoam; Johnson & Johnson, Somerville, New Jersey), acellular cadaveric dermis (Cymetra; LifeCell, Branchburg, New Jersey), calcium hydroxylapatite (Radiesse Voice; Bioform Medical, San Mateo, California), and sodium carboxymethylcellulose aqueous gel (Radiesse Voice Gel; Bioform Medical, San Mateo, Calif., USA). Studies [2, 3] have found a different length of duration for each material (table 1). Teflon has been long abandoned due to risk of granuloma formation.

Some authors have found that children injected with absorbable material will not require a repeat injection. This is thought to be due to a gradual re-lateralization of the vocal fold allowing for adequate compensatory mechanisms to develop [4]. Another possible explanation is that injection of a material may induce fibrosis and scar formation, which increases the bulk of the atrophied vocal fold [3].

Indications

- UVFP
  – Neonate or infant
- Dysphagia
- Recurrent aspiration pneumonia
  – Older children

Table 1. Materials for injection medialization thyroplasty

Product	Material	Duration	Pros	Cons
Gelfoam	bovine gelatin	4–6 weeks	long track record	short effect
Surgifoam	porcine gelatin	4–6 weeks		short effect
Radiesse voice gel	carboxymethylcellulose	2–3 months	no allergy	special needle
Radiesse voice	calcium hydroxylapatite	2–5 years	long effect	special needle
Autologous fat	autologous fat	months to years	no allergy	harvest time
Collagen based				
Zyplast	bovine collagen	4–6 months	long track record	skin testing due to allergy
Cymetra	cadaveric dermis	2–4 months	no allergy	prep. time
Hyaluronic acid gels				
Restalyne	hyaluronic acid bacterial engineered	6–9 months	long effect	stiff
Perlane	hyaluronic acid bacterial engineered	6–9 months	long effect	stiff
Hyalform	hyaluronic acid from rooster combs	6–9 months	long effect	less stiff
Hyalform Plus	hyaluronic acid from rooster combs	6–9 months	long effect	less stiff

Chart from C. Blake Simpson, MD, University of Texas and Albert Mareti, MD, Washington University. Duration represents the length of effect in an adult.

- ◆ Hoarseness
- ◆ Chronic cough
- ◆ Recurrent aspiration pneumonia

- – Glossoptosis
- – Macroglossia
- – Retroflexion of the epiglottis

Contraindications

- Neonates with no evidence of significant dysphagia or aspiration
- – Since the rate of spontaneous recovery for UVFP is high in neonates, it is prudent to wait until a child becomes older prior to performing an injection medialization laryngoplasty. (Injection is performed in neonates with evidence of aspiration or dysphagia to avoid a gastrostomy tube.)
- Poor endoscopic exposure of the larynx
- – Retrognathia
- – Micrognathia

Anesthesia Considerations

- Spontaneous ventilation without intubation
- Intubation
- – Low pulmonary reserve
- – Older children when spontaneous ventilation is not feasible

Preparation

- Modified barium swallow to evaluate swallowing and aspiration
- Laryngeal EMG

- Polyphasic action potentials or any activity
- Consider shorter duration injection material
- No action potentials
- Consider longer duration injectable
- Consider reinnervation procedure
- If there is no etiology for the vocal cord paralysis, an MRI brain and neck looking for any neurologic anomalies should be obtained
- Micro direct laryngoscopy with cricoarytenoid joint palpation
- Special equipment:
- Parsons laryngoscope

Procedure

- Preoperative antibiotics
- Patient positioned in supine position with shoulder roll if necessary
- Spray larynx with 1–4% lidocaine using atomizer
- Parsons laryngoscope placed in vallecula and the patient placed in suspension
- Cut 5.5 endotracheal tube connected to side port of laryngoscope to allow for spontaneous ventilation
- Visualization with Hopkins rod-lens telescope (see online suppl. video 1)
- Injection material (table 1)
- Short-duration short-term paresis/paralysis or in neonates/infants
- Gelfoam (1–1.5 months)
- Surgifoam (1–1.5 months)
- Radiesse voice gel (2–3 months)
- Long duration/long-term paralysis or after failed short-duration injection
- Cymetra (2–4 months)
- Radiesse voice (2–5 years)
- Autologous fat (months to years)
- Injection location
- Lateral to vocal process and lateral to arcuate line (fig. 1)
- Mid-vocal fold, lateral to arcuate line (fig. 2)
- Inject at the glottis medializing the vocal fold

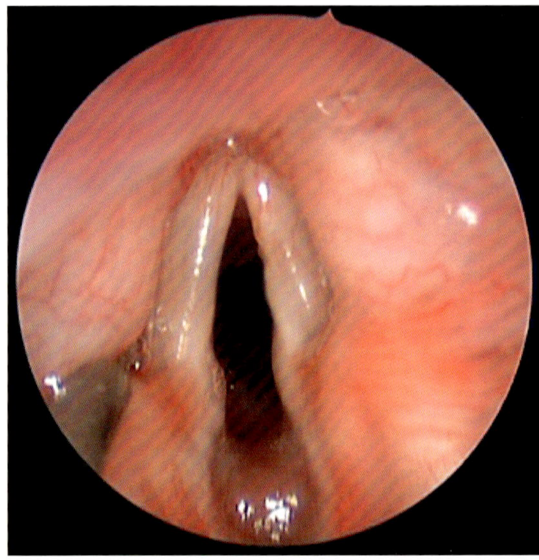

Fig. 1. Preinjection view. Needle is at the first injection point lateral to vocal process and lateral to arcuate line. Note that there is no rotation of the vocal process resulting in a large posterior glottic gap.

- Stop injection when vocal fold is midline
- Inject into the infraglottis medializing conus elasticus
- Helps generate subglottic pressure when vocalizing
- Continually check for infraglottic extension with Hopkins rod telescope
- Injection technique
- 'Stair step' insertion of needle to avoid extravasation of material: enter mucosa; move needle 1–2 mm lateral; push needle in 1–3 mm further
- Suction excess material and reassess (fig. 3)

Postoperative Care

- Admission to PICU (age <1 year) or floor (age >1 year) with continuous pulse oximetry
- Swallow and speech evaluation postoperatively

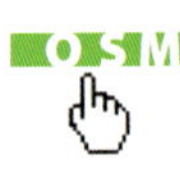

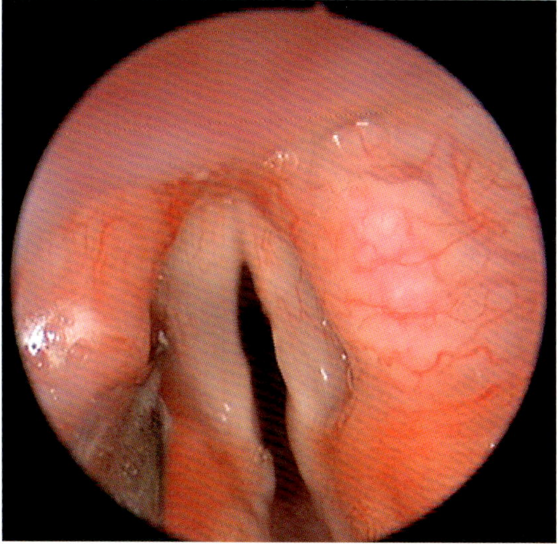

Fig. 2. Needle is at the second injection point lateral to the mid-vocal fold and lateral to the arcuate line.

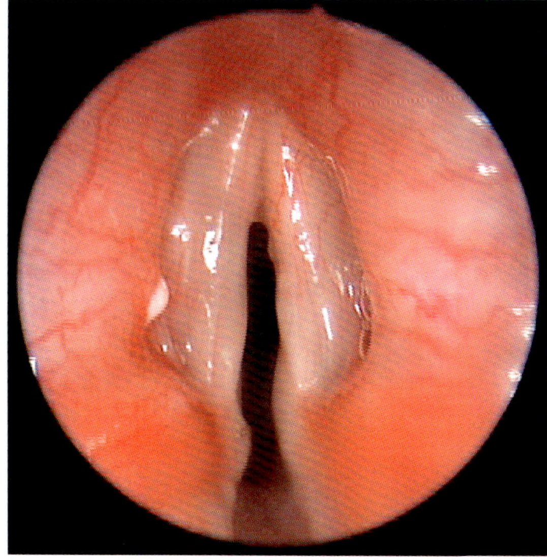

Fig. 3. Postinjection view. Left vocal fold is near midline with some rotation of vocal process.

Pearls

- Continually assess glottic and infraglottic injection with Hopkins rod-lens telescope
- Smooth out injection into vocal fold with straight suction
- Avoid subepithelial injection which will decrease vibratory capacity of vocal fold
  - Remove material if subepithelial injection occurs
- Do not overinject
  - Do not inject so vocal fold is past the midline
  - Do not overaugment conus elasticus

Case Presentation

This was a 2-year-old male with a history of PDA ligation with a hoarse voice, chronic cough, and recurrent aspiration pneumonia. Flexible fiber-optic laryngoscopy was consistent with UVFP. Direct laryngoscopy and bronchoscopy with laryngeal EMG were consistent with good cricoarytenoid joint mobility with no action potentials of the left thyroarytenoid muscle. Left vocal fold injection medialization laryngoplasty was performed. First injection point was lateral to the vocal process and lateral to the arcuate line (fig. 1). Second injection point was lateral to the mid-vocal fold and lateral to the arcuate line (fig. 2). Final view is shown in figure 3.

References

1 Daya H, Hosni A, Bejar-Solar I, Evans JNG, Baily CM: Pediatric vocal fold paralysis: long term prospective study. Arch Otolaryngol Head Neck Surg 2000;126:21–25.

2 Sipp JA, Kerschner JE, Braune N, Hartnick CJ: Vocal fold medialization in children: injection laryngoplasty, thyroplasty, or reinnervation? Arch Otolaryngol Head Neck Surg 2007;133:767–771.

3 Cohen MS, Mehta DK, Maguire RC, Simons JP: Injection medialization in children. Arch Otolaryngol Head Neck Surg 2011;137:264–268.

4 Tucker HM: Vocal cord paralysis in small children: principles in management. Ann Otol Rhinol Laryngol 1986;95:618–621.

Vikash K. Modi, MD, FAAP
Weill Cornell Medical College
Pediatric Otolaryngology, Department of Otolaryngology- Head & Neck Surgery
428 East 72nd Street, Suite 100
New York, NY 10021 (USA)
E-Mail vkm2001@med.cornell.edu

Hartnick CJ, Hansen MC, Gallagher TQ (eds): Pediatric Airway Surgery. Adv Otorhinolaryngol. Basel, Karger, 2012, vol 73, pp 95–100

Laryngeal Cleft

Karen Watters[a] · Lynne Ferrari[b] · Reza Rahbar[a]

Departments of [a]Otolaryngology and Communication Enhancement and [b]Department of Pediatric Anesthesiology, Children's Hospital Boston, Boston, Mass., USA

Abstract

Laryngeal cleft, first described by Richter in 1792, is a rare congenital malformation. Diagnosis can be challenging and is contingent upon a high index of suspicion based on clinical presentation, interpretation of preoperative studies and a thorough endoscopic evaluation under general anesthesia whereby the posterior glottis is carefully palpated for any evidence of a cleft. Management involves feeding and medical therapy. When this fails, endoscopic repair is possible in type 1, 2 and selective type 3 laryngeal clefts. We describe the diagnosis and endoscopic management of type 1 laryngeal clefts, highlighting surgical pearls necessary for success.   Copyright © 2012 S. Karger AG, Basel

Laryngeal cleft is a rare congenital anomaly that is being diagnosed with increased frequency. Incidence is reported as 1 in 10,000 to 1 in 20,000 live births, more common in boys than girls with a ratio of 5:3 [1, 2]. Laryngeal cleft is thought to be a developmental anomaly due to failure of fusion of the tracheoesophageal septum during 5–7th embryonic weeks [3].

Most cases are sporadic. However, in some children the cleft occurs as part of a syndrome, characteristically Opitz-Frias (G) syndrome or Pallister-Hall syndrome. There also appears to be a nonsyndromic association with other airway anomalies (tracheoesophageal fistula, tracheomalacia, laryngomalacia, subglottic stenosis) and anomalies of the cardiac, gastrointestinal,

and genitourinary systems [4, 5]. Nonspecific maternal determinants of risk such as premature delivery, polyhydramnios, and alcohol or drug use during pregnancy have all been reported.

In 1989, Benjamin and Inglis [6] classified laryngeal cleft as 4 types (fig. 1) type 1 – supraglottic interarytenoid defect, in which the cleft lies above the level of the posterior cricoid cartilage; type 2 – cricoid lamina is partially involved with extension below the level of the true vocal cords; type 3 – total cricoid cleft, and type 4 – extends into the posterior wall of the thoracic trachea and may extend as far as the carina.

The diagnosis of type 1 laryngeal cleft can be challenging: presenting symptoms are usually nonspecific and can include feeding difficulty and cough associated with drinking thin liquids, wheeze, chronic cough, and worsening of pulmonary status with upper respiratory tract infections requiring hospital admission [4–7]. Laryngeal cleft should be suspected in any child with a history of recurrent aspiration not attributable to neurologic causes, coughing and choking, post-feed stridor, or strange cry. An early diagnosis of a cleft requires a high level of suspicion and must be looked for on endoscopy by performing specific palpation of the interarytenoid region. Modified swallow studies and fiber-optic endoscopic evaluations of swallowing may be helpful

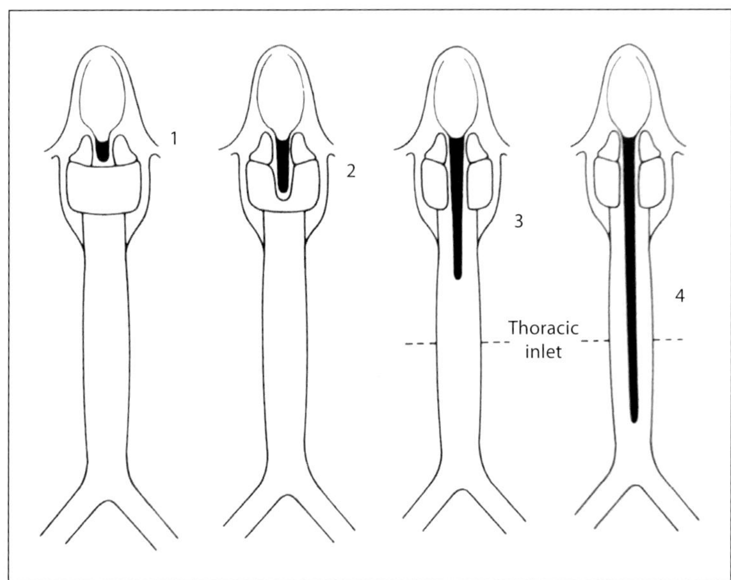

Fig. 1. Benjamin-Inglis Classification System. Reprinted with permisson from [6].

to determine the presence of aspiration; however, a negative study should not exclude a laryngeal cleft [8]. Chest X-rays and CT scans might show pulmonary infiltrates secondary to aspiration. Microlaryngoscopy under general anesthesia remains the gold standard in the diagnosis of laryngeal cleft.

Management of type 1 laryngeal cleft is initially conservative, with feeding therapy, anti-reflux medication, and optimization of respiratory status. Endoscopic repair is possible for type 1, 2, and selective type 3 laryngeal clefts. The open technique is reserved for revision surgery or more extensive clefts. The primary goal of treatment is to minimize respiratory complications related to aspiration and resolve feeding difficulties [7].

Indications

A diagnosis of a type 1 laryngeal cleft alone is not an indication for repair [7].

Factors supporting surgical repair include:
- Poor response to medical management and feeding therapy
- Persistence of aspiration on modified barium swallow
- Findings suggestive of chronic aspiration on chest X-ray or chest CT
- Severity of pulmonary status – recurrent admissions for aspiration-related pneumonias

Contraindications

Relative contraindications include:
- Laryngomalacia or supraglottic airway obstruction – this may worsen following laryngeal cleft repair
- Significant neurologic comorbid conditions predisposing to aspiration
- If endoscopic access or visualization of the posterior glottis is limited, an open approach should be considered

Anesthesia Considerations

- Good communication and preoperative discussion with the anesthesiologist is vital for success

as well as ensuring that the anesthesiologist has a full understanding of the anatomy
- Spontaneous ventilation without an endotracheal tube enables unimpeded visualization and access to the airway for instrumentation, thus eliminating the risk of endotracheal tube-related damage to the suture line
- Anesthesia is best accomplished by inhalation induction (sevoflurane, oxygen, nitrous oxide) followed by administration of intravenous agents (propofol, remifentanil) to maintain unconsciousness. Topical application of 4% (1% and 2% are insufficient) lidocaine to the surgical site for analgesia
- Oxygen can be delivered to the oropharynx using a side port connected to the laryngoscope or through a Venturi needle placed within the lumen of the laryngoscope, and can be reduced during laser use
- Emergency backup ventilation may be provided by a jet ventilator (Sanders) via the Venturi needle or endotracheal intubation and conventional ventilation

Preoperative Preparation

- Laser precautions and safety
- 4% lidocaine for topical laryngeal anesthesia
- Oxymetazoline-soaked ear pledgets to remove excessive char from the laser site and assist hemostasis
- Remove nasogastric oral feeding tube if present

Special Equipment
- Direct laryngobronchoscopy setup including Parsons and Lindholm size-appropriate laryngoscopes
- Laryngeal suspension device (Karl Storz Endoscopy-America Inc.)
- A 10-piece microlaryngeal instrument set, including 3 Kleinsasser endoscopic needle holders, knot pusher (Karl Storz Endoscopy-

America Inc.), small and large alligator forceps, 2 scissors, Lindholm vocal cord retractor (Karl Storz Endoscopy-America Inc.) and Jako probe (Pilling Surgical Instruments; fig. 2)
- Endotracheal tube, in case intubation is necessary
- 0° Hopkins rod 4-mm telescope
- CO_2 laser coupled to an operating microscope with 400-mm lens, focused via a micromanipulator (Carl Zeiss Microimaging Inc.)
- Flexible CO_2 laser fiber (Omniguide, Boston, Mass., USA) for type 3 laryngeal clefts extending into the cervical trachea
- Sutures: 5-0 or 6-0 (for smaller patients) vicryl (polyglactin) on a reverse cutting needle

Surgical Procedure

- Patient supine with shoulder roll to allow mild extension of neck.
- Direct laryngobronchoscopy of the entire upper airway is first performed using a Parson's laryngoscope and a 0° Hopkins rod telescope (online suppl. video 1). The posterior glottis is palpated using a laryngeal probe to confirm the cleft. Any coexisting airway pathology is identified.
- The larynx is visualized with an appropriate-size Lindholm laryngoscope and suspended, ensuring the interarytenoid space is visualized in the center of the microscopic field. In some cases, the vocal cord retractor can be helpful in exposing the entire interarytenoid space [9].
- Topical 4% lidocaine is atomized onto the larynx.
- The mucosal margin of the cleft is denuded using the carbon dioxide laser under microscopic vision at a setting of 3 watts at 0.3-second intermittent mode
- Absorbable interrupted sutures (5-0 or 6-0 vicryl) are then used to close the cleft. Generally, 2–3 sutures are placed, depending

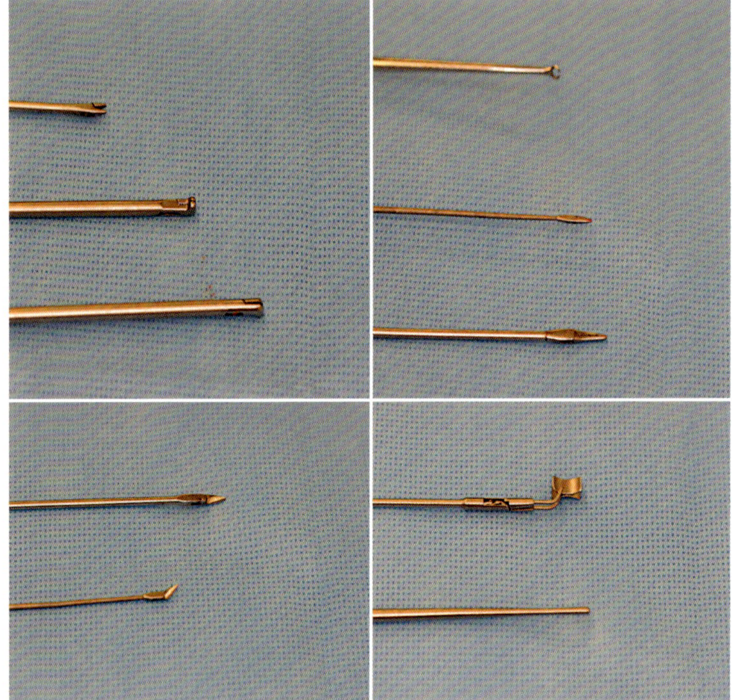

Fig. 2. Ten-piece instrument set consisting of 3 needle holders, stitch pusher, small and large alligator forceps, 2 scissors, vocal cord retractor and a probe.

on the extent of the cleft. Sutures are tied on the posterior surface of the cleft.

- Once the repair is complete, a 0° Hopkins rod telescope is passed into the trachea and blood or secretions that may have pooled are removed. Oropharyngeal secretions are also suctioned.

Postoperative Care

- Admission to the intensive care unit for 24 h, then transferred to the floor for second 24 h
- i.v. antibiotics (ampicillin/sulbactam × 48 h) and i.v. steroids (dexamethasone 0.5 mg/kg × 3 doses) are administered
- Antireflux medication is commenced and continued for 4 weeks
- Preoperative feeding regime is commenced approximately 4 h postoperatively, when the patient is awake and alert

- Discharged on oral antibiotics for 10 days
- Flexible laryngoscopy performed in clinic at 1 week to inspect repair site
- Repeat swallow study in 2–3 months. Alterations in feeding regimes are made at this time.

Pearls

- In confirming the diagnosis of a type 1 laryngeal cleft, excessive force and inferior pressure of the posterior glottis may lead to an incorrect diagnosis
- Adequate endoscopic exposure of the cleft is vital for success – if exposure is limited, an open endoscopic approach should be considered
- It is of paramount importance to completely remove the mucosa at the apex of the cleft to prevent a residual bridge of mucosa with the formation of a fistula at the lower end of the repair

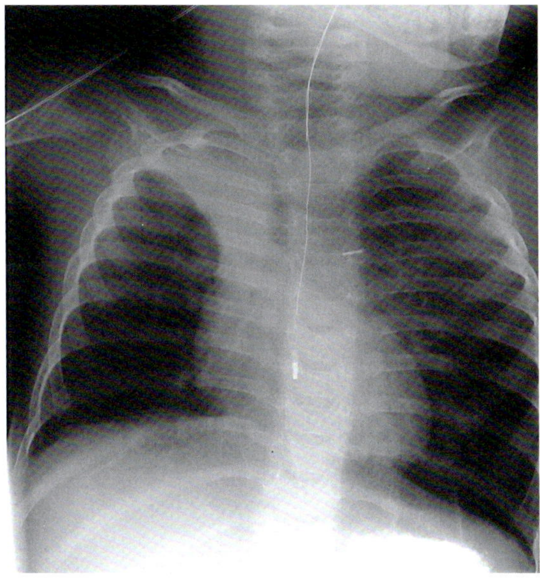

Fig. 3. Chest X-ray showing right upper lobe pneumonia.

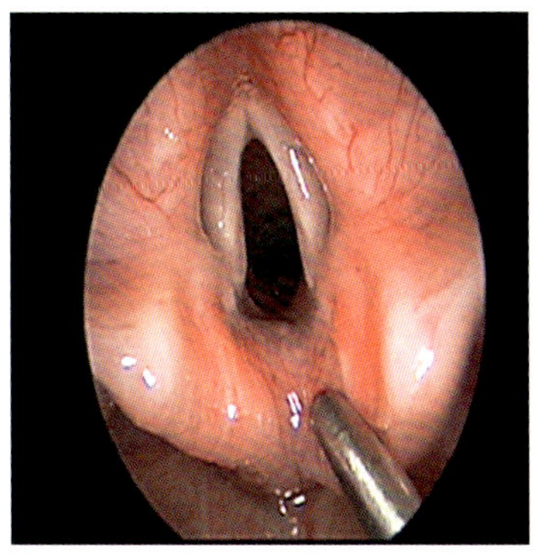

Fig. 4. Type 1 laryngeal cleft identified using a probe on microlaryngoscopy.

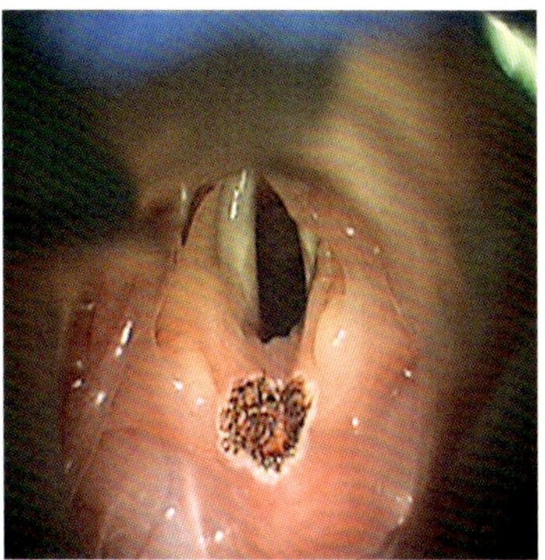

Fig. 5. The mucosa of the cleft is denuded using the carbon dioxide laser.

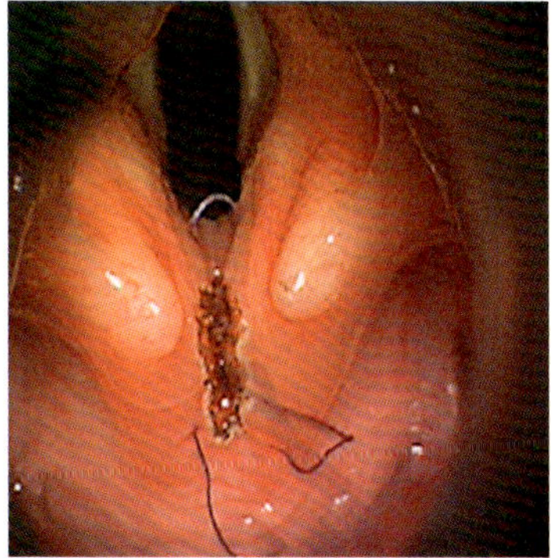

Fig. 6. An absorbable suture is placed in the apex of the cleft.

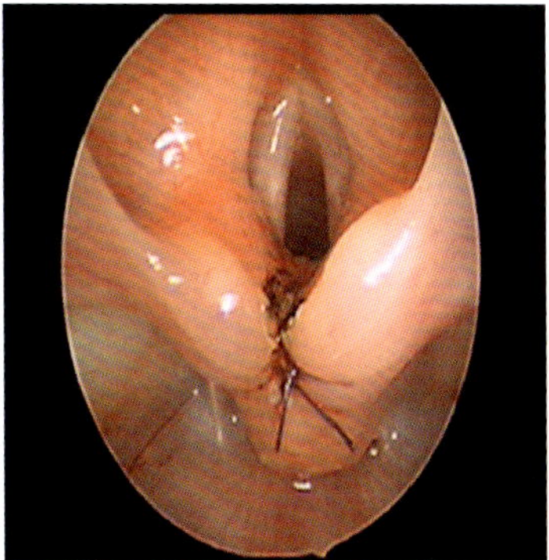

Fig. 7. A second suture is placed and tied posteriorly.

- The first suture is the most important and must be placed at the most inferior extent of the cleft to prevent persistence of a fistula
- When placing sutures, care must be taken not to inadvertently injure healthy mucosa or the epiglottis with the needle tip – this will cause bleeding and make visualization difficult

Case Presentation

This is a 14-month-old male with a history of coughing on drinking fluids and recurrent hospital admissions with lower respiratory tract infections. Chest X-ray showed evidence of right upper lobe opacification consistent with pneumonia secondary to aspiration (fig. 3). A type 1 laryngeal cleft was diagnosed on direct microlaryngobronchoscopy (fig. 4). No other airway anomalies were identified. Endoscopic repair of type 1 laryngeal cleft was performed. Carbon dioxide laser was used to denude mucosa of cleft (fig. 5). A 5-0 vicryl suture was placed in the apex of the cleft (fig. 6). A second suture was placed and tied on the posterior surface (fig. 7).

References

1 Richter CF: Dissertatio medico de infanticide inartis obstetriciae; thesis, Leipzig, 1792.
2 Roth B, Rose KG, Benz-Bohm G, Gunther H: Laryngotracheoesophageal cleft: clinical features, diagnosis and therapy. Eur J Pediatr 1983;140:41–46.
3 Delahunty JE, Cherry J: Congenital laryngeal clefts. Ann Otol Rhinol Laryngol 1969;78:96–106.
4 Watters K, Russell J: Diagnosis and management of type 1 laryngeal cleft. Int J Pediatr Otorhinolaryngol 2003;67:591–596.
5 Rahbar R, Rouillon I, Rogers G, et al: The presentation and management of laryngeal cleft: a 10-year experience. Arch Otolaryngol Head Neck Surg 2006;132:1335–1341.
6 Benjamin B, Inglis A: Minor congenital laryngeal clefts: diagnosis and classification. Ann Otol Rhinol Laryngol 1989;98:417–420.
7 Rahbar R, Chen JL, Rosen RL, Lowry KC, Simon DM, Perez JA, Buonomo C, Ferrari LR, Katz ES: Endoscopic repair of laryngeal cleft type 1 and type 2: when and why? Laryngoscope 2009;119:1797–1802.
8 Chien W, Ashland J, Haver K, Hardy SC, Curren P, Hartnick CJ: Type 1 laryngeal cleft: establishing a functional diagnostic and management algorithm. Int J Pediatr Otorhinolaryngol 2006;70:2073–2079.
9 Maturo S, Hartnick CJ: The vocal fold retractor: a useful tool for diagnosis and treatment of laryngeal and tracheal pathology. Laryngoscope 2010;120:2227–2230.

Karen Watters
Department of Otolaryngology and Communication Enhancement
Children's Hospital Boston, 300 Longwood Avenue, LO-367
Boston, MA 02115 (USA)
E-Mail karen.watters@childrens.harvard.edu

Hartnick CJ, Hansen MC, Gallagher TQ (eds): Pediatric Airway Surgery. Adv Otorhinolaryngol. Basel, Karger, 2012, vol 73, pp 101–104

Pediatric Supraglottoplasty

Art Ambrosio · Matthew T. Brigger

Department of Otolaryngology, Head and Neck Surgery, Naval Medical Center San Diego, San Diego, Calif., USA

Abstract

Laryngomalacia is the most common congenital laryngeal abnormality, as well as the most common cause of stridor in infants. Laryngomalacia presents as a wide spectrum of disease from mild noisy breathing with feeding to life-threatening airway obstruction and failure to thrive. The stridor associated with laryngomalacia is generally inspiratory in nature from supraglottic airway collapse. Supraglottoplasty refers to a group of procedures used for the surgical management of laryngomalacia. In this chapter, the authors review laryngomalacia and describe the surgical techniques of supraglottoplasty.

Laryngomalacia is the most common congenital laryngeal abnormality as well as the most common cause of stridor in infants. Laryngomalacia results from dynamic airway obstruction originating from abnormal supraglottic structures [1, 2]. Laryngomalacia presents as a wide spectrum of disease from mild noisy breathing with feeding to life-threatening airway obstruction and failure to thrive. Anatomic configurations are variable

and include redundant arytenoid mucosa ('floppers'), short aryepiglottic folds ('curlers') with retroflexion of the epiglottis or a combination of both.

A postulated theory of etiology is that laryngeal tone and sensorimotor integrative function of the larynx is fundamentally altered in affected children [3]. The degree of alteration correlates with disease severity, indicating that factors that alter the peripheral and central pathways of the laryngeal adductor reflex have a role in the etiology of signs and symptoms of laryngomalacia. The presence of Gastroesophageal reflux disease (GERD), neurologic disease, and low Apgar scores are associated with increasing disease severity. Sensorimotor integrative function is noted to improve as symptoms resolve [3].

Regardless of etiology, GERD has been well documented in association with laryngomalacia, with worsening of laryngeal edema subsequently worsening respiratory symptoms [4, 5]. Evaluation of GERD should take place in the preoperative setting and the effect of medical management determined prior to surgery.

The diagnosis of laryngomalacia includes a detailed history of the description of the stridor, cyanotic/apneic events, exacerbating factors, as well as its association with feeding. The stridor associated with laryngomalacia is generally inspiratory in nature from supraglottic airway collapse. Further, physical examination should initially evaluate the infant's work of breathing and must include awake fiberoptic flexible laryngoscopy to evaluate for dynamic supraglottic collapse and its causative factors [6]. Polysomnography may prove useful in some children, particularly in the setting of neurologic disease. Children with evidence of dysphagia, particularly when aspiration symptoms are reported should undergo a detailed swallowing evaluation with video fluoroscopic evaluation or functional endoscopic evaluation of swallowing.

Indications

- Failure to thrive, weight loss, or significant feeding difficulty
- Recurrent cyanotic events
- Obstructive apnea
- Secondary cardiopulmonary pathology such as pulmonary hypertension or cor pulmonale

Contraindications

None.

Anesthesia Considerations

General anesthesia is given with spontaneous ventilation or endotracheal intubation based on surgeon preference and degree of pulmonary reserve.

Preparation

- Preoperative
- Symptoms are monitored through a trial of anti-reflux therapy and thickening of feeds
- Consideration of a polysomnogram
- Flexible fiber-optic laryngoscopic video is reviewed to plan operative strategy
- Intraoperative

– Dexamethasone i.v. is given at 0.5 mg/kg
– Direct laryngoscopy is performed to bring supraglottic anatomy into view, followed by bronchoscopy to evaluate for synchronous airway lesions
– The surgical procedure is tailored to specific anatomic issues identified on preoperative flexible laryngoscopy. Specific interventions include:
- Excision of redundant arytenoids mucosa for 'floppers'. Specific methods include powered microdebrider, CO_2/KTP laser, cold micro-laryngeal instruments.
- Division of the tight aryepiglottic folds in 'curlers'. Specific methods include cold microlaryngeal instruments (author's preference), powered microdebrider, or CO_2/KTP laser

Procedure

- The child is placed into laryngeal suspension with an operating laryngoscope (Lindholm preferred by the senior author)
- The child is maintained in a plane of spontaneous breathing anesthesia or a small-caliber endotracheal tube is placed
- An operating microscope or 0° Hopkins rod telescope is used for intraoperative magnification.
- For redundant mucosa associated with arytenoid prolapse, ablation with a CO_2 laser or resection with a 2.9-mm laryngeal skimmer blade is employed for controlled, sequential removal (see online suppl. video 1).
- Aryepiglottic fold division is used via microlaryngeal scissors or CO_2/KTP laser (see online suppl. video 2).
- Intraoperative countertraction for visualization may be performed by gentle use of microlaryngeal forceps or a straight laryngeal suction.
- Epinephrine-soaked pledgets are utilized as necessary for hemostasis.

- If a laser-based technique is utilized, laser safety precautions for both the patient and the operating room staff including covering the child's face/eyes with moist towels/eye pads are essential

Postoperative Care

- The child may be extubated immediately or on postoperative day one with admission to the Pediatric ICU for continuous respiratory monitoring
- Decadron 0.5 mg/kg is given every 8 h for 24 h.
- Restart anti-reflux medication, thickened feeds, and anti-reflux precautions (e.g. head of bed elevation, keeping of infant upright after feeds for a period of 30–40 min)
- Antibiotic coverage for a period of 7–10 days is recommended

Complications

- Potential complications include supraglottic stenosis, persistent feeding difficulties including aspiration, persistent airway obstruction or laser-specific issues such as airway fires
- Postoperatively, transient new-onset aspiration has been reported to occur in up to 28% of children [7]. Such aspiration seldom requires more than a brief period of thickening the feeds.

Pearls

- Laryngomalacia is the most common cause of stridor in the newborn; the choice of a tailored supraglottoplasty in a select population can have a profound effect in respiratory effort and feeding
- A trial of anti-reflux medication and precautions will help to delineate nonoperative from operative candidates in the preoperative evaluation.
- Surgical intervention is based on a targeted approach derived from a dynamic evaluation of supraglottic collapse.
- Maintaining postoperative anti-reflux therapy is recommended.
- A directed sufficient, but not overzealous resection of tissue is important to alleviate symptoms, but not cause supraglottic stenosis. Unilateral supraglottoplasty has been advocated to avoid postoperative supraglottic scarring. In the author's experience, judicious resection bilaterally has proven safe and maximally effective.
- Judicious supraglottoplasty is associated with few complications and clinical improvement in >85% of children undergoing the procedure [3, 7, 8]
- Excellent results can be obtained regardless of surgical modality (cold instruments, laser) provided the surgical approach is well thought out. Selection of modality is based on surgeon preference and experience
- Laser safety precautions and closed-loop communication during oxygen titration are paramount when lasers are used

Case Presentation

A 3-month-old male, otherwise healthy, term-infant, was followed since his 2nd day of life for progressively worsening inspiratory stridor. By the sixth week of life, the child had developed feeding difficulties and interruption secondary to respiratory difficulty with resultant poor weight gain. His physical examination was significant for inspiratory stridor worsening with agitation. Fiber-optic flexible laryngoscopy revealed an omega-shaped epiglottis, short aryepiglottic folds, and dynamic collapse of the supraglottis into the laryngeal inlet. The patient had continued symptoms with cyanotic episodes that self-resolved, as well as poor weight gain despite an anti-reflux regimen including thickened feeds and maximal proton pump inhibitor therapy. A modified barium swallow demonstrated no evidence of aspiration. Given the progressive symptoms and failure to thrive, the family was offered operative intervention. Direct laryngoscopy and bronchoscopy confirmed findings of an omega-shaped epiglottis, short aryepiglottic folds, and no evidence of a secondary airway lesion such as subgottic stenosis or tracheobronchomalacia. Suspension laryngoscopy was performed with a Lindholm laryngoscope following completion of the bronchoscopy, and adequate spontaneous ventilation anesthesia was obtained. Aryepiglottic fold division was performed bilaterally using microlaryngeal scissors. The author judiciously removed triangular wedges of the aryepiglottic folds. The patient's postoperative course was uneventful with immediate improvement in stridor and feeding. At the 6-week postoperative visit, the child demonstrated appropriate weight gain, no clinical evidence of aspiration and minimal inspiratory stridor. The parents voiced a high level of satisfaction.

References

1 Richter GT, Thompson DM: The surgical management of laryngomalacia. Otolaryngol Clin North Am 2008;41:837–864, vii.
2 Zoumalan R, Maddalozzo J, Holinger LD: Etiology of stridor in infants. Ann Otol Rhinol Laryngol 2007;116:329–334.
3 Thompson DM: Abnormal sensorimotor integrative function of the larynx in congenital laryngomalacia: a new theory of etiology. Laryngoscope 2007;117:1–33.
4 Messner AH: Congenital Disorders of the Larynx. Cummings Otolaryngology: Head & Neck Surgery, ed 5. Philadelphia, Mosby, 2010.
5 Matthews BL, Little JP, McGuirt WF, et al: Reflux in infants with laryngomalacia: results of 24-hour double-probe pH monitoring. Otolaryngol Head Neck Surg 1999;120:860–864.
6 Solomons NB, Prescott CA: Laryngomalacia. A review and the surgical management for severe cases. Intl J Pediatric Otorhinolaryngol 1987;13:31–39.
7 Schroeder JW Jr, Thakkar KH, Poznanovic SA, Holinger LD: Aspiration following CO_2 laser-assisted supraglottoplasty. Int J Pediatr Otorhinolaryngol 2008;72: 985–990.
8 Denoyelle F, Mondain M, Gresillon N, Roger G, Chaudre F, Garabedian EN: Failures and complications of supraglottoplasty in children. Arch Otolaryngol Head Neck Surg 2003;129:1077–1080.

Matthew T. Brigger, MD, MPH, LCDR, MC, USN
Naval Medical Center San Diego
Department of Otolaryngology, Head and Neck Surgery
34800 Bob Wilson Drive
San Diego, CA 92134 (USA)
E-Mail matthew.brigger@med.navy.mil

Hartnick CJ, Hansen MC, Gallagher TQ (eds): Pediatric Airway Surgery. Adv Otorhinolaryngol. Basel, Karger, 2012, vol 73, pp 105–108

Juvenile-Onset Recurrent Respiratory Papillomatosis

Stephen C. Maturo[a] · Christopher J. Hartnick[b]

[a]Department of Otolaryngology, San Antonio Military Medical Center, Fort Sam Houston, Tex.,
[b]Department of Otology and Laryngology, Massachusetts Eye & Ear Infirmary, Boston, Mass., USA

Abstract

Juvenile-onset recurrent respiratory papillomatosis, caused by the human papilloma virus, is the most common benign neoplasm of the larynx in children. Recurrent respiratory papillomatosis is relatively rare, but it can have a significant impact on afflicted children and their family's quality of life as dysphonia and multiple surgical procedures are hallmarks of this disease. The current standard of care is surgical therapy with a goal of complete papilloma removal and preservation of normal structures. The technique in this atlas combines both the microdebrider and the pulse KTP laser. The microdebrider allows for rapid removal of bulky lesions without the risk of thermal injury, yet it cannot provide precise removal in areas such as the anterior commissure and ventricle. The pulse KTP laser allows for removal of sessile lesions and in sensitive areas such as the vocal folds. The authors describe this technique as well as discuss adjuvant therapies and pearls for success.

The views expressed in this article are those of the authors and do not necessarily reflect the official policy or position of the Department of the Air Force, Department of Defense, or the United States Government.

Stephen C. Maturo is a military service member. This work was prepared as part of his official duties. Title 17 .S.C. 105 provides that 'Copyright protection under this title is not available for any work of the United States Government.' Title 17 U.S.C. 101 defines a United States Government work as a work prepared by a military service member or employee of the United States Government as part of that person's official duties.

Juvenile-onset recurrent respiratory papillomatosis (JORRP; see online suppl. video 1), caused by 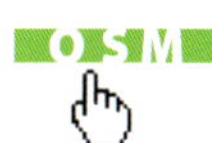 the human papilloma virus (HPV), is the most common benign neoplasm of the larynx in children [1]. It is most commonly caused by HPV types 6 and 11, although types 16 and 18 can also be found, and these types raise the concern about possible malignant transformation [2–4]. Recurrent respiratory papillomatosis (RRP) is relatively rare, but it can have a significant impact on afflicted children and their family's quality of life as dysphonia and multiple surgical procedures are hallmarks of this disease [2, 5]. Although it is a benign disease, RRP can recur often and can cause frank airway obstruction; moreover, there is the concern about malignant conversion. There is also growing concern about the effect of multiple anesthetics in the developing child in terms of behavior changes and possible learning delays [6, 7].

The current standard of care is surgical therapy with a goal of complete papilloma removal and preservation of normal structures. This requires a fine balance between meticulous papilloma removal resulting in an increased interval between procedures and avoiding injury to the developing vocal fold in order to ensure optimal voice outcomes. Surgical therapy has been the mainstay of treatment of RRP, but adjuvant medical therapies have been administered with overall mixed results [8–12]. Unlike adult RRP treatment that is now commonly performed in a clinic setting, management of children requires a trip to the operating room. Surgical techniques may consist of cold knife endolaryngeal incision with or without phonosurgical technique, excision with the microdebrider (Medtronic, Minneapolis, Minn., USA), carbon dioxide, pulsed dye or 532 pulsed KTP lasers or a combination of these techniques. The technique in this atlas combines both the microdebrider and the pulse KTP laser. The microdebrider allows for rapid removal of bulky lesions without the risk of thermal injury, yet it cannot provide precise removal in areas such as the anterior commissure and ventricle. The pulse KTP laser allows for removal of sessile lesions and in sensitive areas such as the vocal folds. The pulse KTP laser provides a longer thermal relaxation time when compared to the CO_2 and PDL laser with the resulting theoretical benefit of reduced thermal injury to the lamina propria. With the recent development of the HPV vaccine, there is hope that RRP will be eradicated in future generations, but until that time there will continue to be a need in a subset of individuals for adjuvant therapy that can prevent additional surgeries and improve quality of life [2–5, 8–12]. Although no standard exists, it is recommended that adjuvant therapy such as intralesional cidofovir (Gilead Sciences, USA) injection be considered when children require more than 4 surgical treatments per year. Finally, when considering adjuvant therapy, separate informed consents are recommended that specifically discuss the rare but documented side effects of these medications.

Indications

- Child with suspected JORRP needing pathologic diagnosis and airway evaluation
- Child with known JORRP having airway symptoms

Contraindications

None.

Preoperative Preparation

- Determine urgency of treatment based on airway symptoms
- Possible chest X-ray or computed tomography scan if concern for pulmonary spread
- If considering adjuvant therapy, then extensive pretreatment counseling is necessary. Risks, benefits, and alternative therapies need to be discussed and documented fully.
- For older children diagnosed with new-onset JORRP one must consider evaluation for sexual exposure/abuse

Anesthesia Considerations

- An experienced anesthesiologist is necessary
- Spontaneous ventilation is optimal, but apneic technique is possible
- Topical lidocaine is applied to the laryngeal structures. 4% lidocaine is typically used being mindful of the maximum dosage allowed based on the child's weight.
- If a laser is used, close coordination with the anesthesiologist is necessary to prevent airway fires
- Appropriate measures should be taken for smoke evacuation during the laser procedure

Equipment Needed

- Operating microscope
- Suspension laryngoscopy
- Microlaryngeal instruments
- Microdebrider with various cutting blades
- Desired laser

- Lindholm vocal cord and false cord retractor (Karl Storz, Germany) is a useful instrument to help visualize the vocal folds while removing papilloma [13] (see online suppl. video 2)
- Afrin soaked pledgets

Surgical Procedure

- Once the appropriate level of anesthesia is obtained, the child is placed in suspension
- Topical lidocaine (4%) is applied via an atomizer to the larynx being mindful of the maximum dosage limits based on the child's weight
- If a laser is to be used, appropriate precautions to include moist eye pads and moist towels applied to child's exposed skin are necessary
- Biopsy specimens are taken as warranted
- Described technique uses a combination of microdebrider (see online suppl. video 3) for efficiently addressing bulky disease and the pulsed KTP laser (see online suppl. video 4) for addressing the vocal folds, ventricle and smaller, sessile lesions. The pulse KTP laser provides the theoretical advantage of selective photoangiolysis with a longer relaxation time, which helps preserve the important layered structures of the vocal fold.
- If adjuvant therapy is required, it is injected into the areas most significantly affected by papilloma (see online suppl. video 5)
- We use adjuvant therapy on a regularly scheduled bi-weekly basis over an 8- to 10-week period
- If results are not seen by 12 weeks, then consideration is given to a stopping of the adjuvant therapy or trying a new adjuvant therapy

Postoperative Care

- Depending on clinical scenario, the child can be observed overnight or discharged home 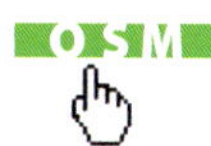
- Review pathology results to ensure diagnosis and HPV subtyping
- Yearly biopsy specimen should be considered if suspicious changes to evaluate for malignant degeneration

Pearls

- Using the Derkay staging system during each trip to the operating room allows for an accurate comparison and analysis of treatment results
- Extreme diligence needs to be taken when operating near the anterior commissure. Consider only addressing one anterior vocal fold at each session to avoid anterior webs or scars. 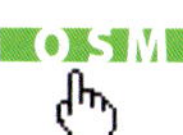
- The pulse KTP laser is NOT a contact laser and works best when placed approximately 1–2 mm away from intended target
- An effective technique includes using a suction to 'wipe' away the char formed after a few passes with the laser
- Once a pattern for recurrence is established, caregivers can be counseled to return as symptoms warrant. It should be stressed that caregivers should not wait until significant worsening of symptoms so as to prevent respiratory embarrassment.

References

1 Derkay CS, Wiatrak B: Recurrent respiratory papillomatosis: a review. Laryngoscope 2008;118:1236–1247.

2 Reeves WC, et al: National registry for juvenile-onset recurrent respiratory papillomatosis. Arch Otolaryngol Head Neck Surg 2003;129:976–982.

3 Rosen CA, Bryson PC: Indole-3-carbinol for recurrent respiratory papillomatosis: long-term results. J Voice 2004;18:248–253.

4   Rosen CA, et al: Preliminary results of the use of indole-3-carbinol for recurrent respiratory papillomatosis. Otolaryngol Head Neck Surg 1998;118:810–815.

5   Snoeck R, et al: Treatment of severe laryngeal papillomatosis with intralesional injections of cidofovir [(S)-1-(3-hydroxy-2-phosphonylmethoxypropyl)cytosine]. J Med Virol 1998;54:219–225.

6   Kalkman CJ, et al: Behavior and development in children and age at the time of first anesthetic exposure. Anesthesiology 2009;110:805–812.

7   Wilder RT, et al: Early exposure to anesthesia and learning disabilities in a population-based birth cohort. Anesthesiology 2009;110:796–804.

8   Pransky SM, et al: Clinical update on 10 children treated with intralesional cidofovir injections for severe recurrent respiratory papillomatosis. Arch Otolaryngol Head Neck Surg 2000;126:1239–1243.

9   Pransky SM, et al: Intralesional cidofovir for recurrent respiratory papillomatosis in children. Arch Otolaryngol Head Neck Surg 1999;125:1143–1148.

10 Pashley NR: Can mumps vaccine induce remission in recurrent respiratory papilloma? Arch Otolaryngol Head Neck Surg 2002;128:783–786.

11 Maturo S, Tse SM, Kinane B, Hartnick CJ: Initial experience using propranolol as adjunctive treatment in children with aggressive respiratory papillomatosis. Ann Otol Rhinol Laryngol 2011;120:17–20.

12 Maturo S, Hartnick C: Use of 532-nm pulsed potassium titanyl phosphate laser and adjuvant intralesional bevacizumab for aggressive respiratory papillomatosis in children: initial experience. Arch Otolaryngol Head Neck Surg 2010;136:561–565.

13 Maturo S, Hartnick CJ: The vocal fold retractor: a useful tool for diagnosis and treatment of laryngeal and tracheal pathology. Laryngoscope 2010;120:2227–2230.

Christopher J. Hartnick, MD
Professor, Department of Otology and Laryngology
Chief, Division of Pediatric Otolaryngology
Director, Pediatric Airway, Voice and Swallowing Center
Chief Quality Officer
Massachusetts Eye and Ear Infirmary, Harvard Medical School
243 Charles Street
Boston, MA 02116 (USA)
E-Mail christopher_hartnick@meei.harvard.edu

Hartnick CJ, Hansen MC, Gallagher TQ (eds): Pediatric Airway Surgery. Adv Otorhinolaryngol. Basel, Karger, 2012, vol 73, pp 109–111

Pediatric Lingual Tonsillectomy

Stephen C. Maturo[a] · Christopher J. Hartnick[b]

[a]Department of Otolaryngology, San Antonio Military Medical Center, Fort Sam Houston, Tex.,
[b]Department of Otology and Laryngology, Massachusetts Eye & Ear Infirmary, Boston, Mass., USA

Abstract

Tonsillectomy and adenoidectomy are an effective surgical treatment of pediatric obstructive sleep apnea; however, up to 20% of these patients can have persistent disease. In this select patient population, the lingual tonsil may be an occult source of obstruction. Lingual tonsillectomy can be a challenging procedure due to poor access and visualization, airway edema, postoperative pain and hemostasis during tissue removal. In this chapter, we describe our preferred technique for lingual tonsillectomy including surgical pearls for success.

Sleep-disordered breathing is one of the more common entities seen by pediatric otolaryngologists. Tonsillectomy and adenoidectomy are a successful surgical treatment for children with obstructive sleep apnea (OSA) due to tonsil and adenoid hypertrophy. Yet, 10–20% of children have persistent OSA following tonsillectomy and adenoidectomy [1].

The views expressed in this article are those of the authors and do not necessarily reflect the official policy or position of the Department of the Air Force, Department of Defense, or the United States Government.

Stephen C. Maturo is a military service member. This work was prepared as part of his official duties. Title 17 .S.C. 105 provides that 'Copyright protection under this title is not available for any work of the United States Government.' Title 17 U.S.C. 101 defines a United States Government work as a work prepared by a military service member or employee of the United States Government as part of that person's official duties.

One of the more common overlooked sites for continued obstruction is lingual tonsil hypertrophy. Historically, lingual tonsillectomy has been a challenge due to poor access and visualization, airway edema, postoperative pain and hemostasis during tissue removal. Various techniques have been described with many involving suspension laryngoscopy for access. Instruments for tissue removal have included suction electrocautery, laser, and microdebrider (Medtronic, Minneapolis, Minn., USA). Robinson et al. [2] reported on use of coblation (Arthrocare, Austin, Tex., USA) with suspension laryngoscopy in 2006 touting better exposure, faster dissection, better visualization, and improved hemostasis. Despite these benefits, we find the laryngoscope cumbersome, bulky and needing frequent readjustments. Transitioning to a direct endoscopic technique employing otolaryngic skills from sinus surgery and airway endoscopy and utilizing coblation, lingual tonsillectomy has become significantly easier procedure to perform [3].

In this chapter, we describe an endoscopic technique using readily available equipment that may overcome access limitations of previously described techniques while also providing a more thorough removal of offending tissue [3].

Indications

Lingual tonsil hypertrophy resulting in sleep-disordered breathing or other symptomatic airway issues.

Contraindications

Similar to those of tonsillectomy.

Preoperative Preparation

- Awake flexible fiber-optic endoscopy is recommended to diagnose lingual tonsil hypertrophy
- Other methods to evaluate upper airway obstruction involving the lingual tonsils include sleep/sedated fluoroscopy, sedated cine MRI and intraoperative sedated endoscopy
- MRI is able to distinguish between lingual tonsil tissue and base of tongue musculature
- Cine MRI comes from the French word ciné, short for cinema. It records a series of sequential magnetic resonance pictures, creating a 'movie' (hence the term 'cine'), of the upper airway during sleep, and can help define the location of upper airway obstruction.

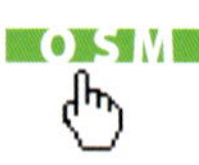

- The authors use cine MRI in cases of severe OSA status after adenotonsillectomy where the patient will not tolerate any medical management (i.e. continuous positive airway pressure mask) or if there is clinical suspicion for lingual tonsillar obstruction based on examination
- Cine MRI requires sedation
- Sedation for the above procedures can involve use of propofol/remifentanil infusion with zero end-tidal inhalational agent [4] or dexmedetomidine. Regardless of the choice of anesthetic, the goal is to monitor the degree of sedation in hopes of mimicking sleep in order to identify the site of obstruction.

Anesthesia Considerations

- Nasotracheal intubation
- Intravenous dexamethasone (0.5 mg/kg, max. dose of 10 mg)
- Intraoperative antibiotics are not routinely administered

Equipment Needed

- 2.0 silk suture
- Bite Block, Medesey mouth gag (aka 'side biter' mouth gag), or Jennings mouth gag
- Red rubber catheters to elevate the palate are optional
- 30° and 70° rigid endoscope with camera and video tower
- Coblator EVac 70 coblation wand (Arthrocare ENT, Austin, Tex., USA)
- Coblation setting of 8 and a coagulation setting of 5

Surgical Procedure

- Once nasotracheal intubation has been performed, a 2.0 silk suture is placed in the midline of the anterior tongue to aid in retraction (see online suppl. video 1)
- An appropriately sized mouth gag or bite block is placed
- Red rubber catheters are placed through the nose to retract the soft palate
- The surgeon stands at the head of the bed with a video tower to the right
- The assistant aids the surgeon by retracting the anterior placed tongue stitch
- Significant retraction is often required
- With the aid of the endoscope, the coblation wand is used as a blunt dissector to identify the uvula and the base of the vallecula
- To avoid blood contaminating the endoscope, it is best to work from the base of the tongue

in an anterior-superior direction towards the circumvallate papilla

- The lingual tonsils are removed sequentially
- Any bleeding is addressed with the coagulation setting of the coblator
- Once a satisfactory amount of obstructing tissue is removed, the tongue stitch is removed and the patient is extubated

Postoperative Care

- Postoperative observation in a monitored setting is appropriate
- We use the same protocol as done for tonsillectomy to determine whether the patient can be monitored on a regular floor bed or if a higher level of care is necessary
- Routine postoperative antibiotics are not administered
- Pain control regimens are similar to those after tonsillectomy
- There does not seem to be increased pain in this procedure when compared to a standard tonsillectomy
- Parents should be warned about appropriate oral intake and postoperative bleeding
- A repeat postoperative polysomnogram is recommended no earlier than 6 weeks after surgery

- Concerns for reflux or allergies should be considered if regrowth of lingual tonsil tissue occurs after an adequate removal
- The tongue base musculature may still be the offending upper airway site of obstruction after adequate lingual tonsil removal and may need to be addressed at a future time

Pearls

- Retraction with the silk suture will provide more visualization and allow for more complete removal
- Always have the coblation wand facing the tongue base to avoid injury to the lingual surface of the epiglottis and posterior pharyngeal wall
- When working inferiorly, the epiglottis should be kept in view at all times in order to prevent inadvertent damage
- Remain cognizant of how far lateral the dissection proceeds
- In some children, you may notice a pulsating internal carotid artery which should serve as a reminder
- Enlarged lingual tonsils may cause an obscured airway on intubation, and it may be worthwhile to be present during intubation during these cases

References

1 Lin A, Koltai P: Persistent pediatric obstructive sleep apnea and lingual tonsillectomy. Otolaryngol Head Neck Surg 2009;141:81–85.

2 Robinson S, Ettema SL, Brusky L, et al: Lingual tonsillectomy using bipolar radiofrequency plasma excision. Otolaryngol Head Neck Surg 2006;134:328–330.

3 Maturo SC, Mair EA: Coblation lingual tonsillectomy. Otolaryngol Head Neck Surg 2006;135:487–488.

4 Thevasagayam M, Rodger K, Cave D, Williams M, El-Hakim H: Prevalence of laryngogomalacia in children with sleep-disordered breathing. Laryngoscope 2010;120:1662–1666.

Christopher J. Hartnick, MD
Professor, Department of Otology and Laryngology
Chief, Division of Pediatric Otolaryngology
Director, Pediatric Airway, Voice and Swallowing Center
Chief Quality Officer, Massachusetts Eye and Ear Infirmary, Harvard Medical School
243 Charles Street
Boston, MA 02116 (USA)
E-Mail christopher_hartnick@meei.harvard.edu

Hartnick CJ, Hansen MC, Gallagher TQ (eds): Pediatric Airway Surgery. Adv Otorhinolaryngol. Basel, Karger, 2012, vol 73, pp 112–115

Pediatric Airway Balloon Dilation

Stephen C. Maturo[a] · Christopher J. Hartnick[b]

[a]Department of Otolaryngology, San Antonio Military Medical Center, Fort Sam Houston, Tex.,
[b]Department of Otology and Laryngology, Massachusetts Eye & Ear Infirmary, Boston, Mass., USA

Abstract

Over the past decade, there has also been renewed interest in serial dilatation for the management of subglottic and tracheal stenosis with the advent of new technologies such as airway balloons designed for the pediatric airway. In this chapter, the authors describe the technique of application of airway balloons as a useful adjunct for management of airway lesions.

Over the past decade, there has been a renaissance in the use of endoscopic procedures in the management of airway lesions with the rising notoriety of procedures such as endoscopic cleft repair and endoscopic posterior cricoid graft laryngoplasty. There has also been renewed interest in serial dilatation for the management of subglottic and tracheal stenosis with the advent of new technologies such as airway balloons designed for the pediatric airway [1]. The purpose of this chapter is not to debate the merits of endoscopic dilatation versus open reconstruction or resection, but rather to describe the application of airway balloons as a useful adjunct for management of airway lesions.

The main theoretical advantage of airway balloons over rigid dilatation includes the balloon's radial, non-shearing force which allows for a more gentle and precise dilatation [1–3]. Also, with the small size of airway balloons they can be easily visualized with current rigid endoscopes during the entire procedure. Disadvantages of airway balloons are their cost and the absence of prospective trials demonstrating a worthwhile advantage. At the Massachusetts Eye and Ear Infirmary airway, balloons are most commonly used during the initial endoscopic evaluations after laryngotracheal reconstruction to release any early scar and to help gently dilate the swollen subglottis as the healing process continues over the first 2–4 weeks. This chapter focuses on the laryngotracheal application of airway balloons, but one would be remiss to not mention their rising popularity in sinus disease management [4]. Airway balloons have also been applied to eustachian tube lesions and choanal stenosis [5, 6].

Indications

- Glottic, subglottic, tracheal stenosis as initial management
- Postoperative dilatation after open laryngotracheal reconstruction

- Salvage management of laryngotracheal reconstruction
- Sinus management, choanal atresia, and nasopharyngeal stenosis

Contraindications

- Early application after cricotracheal or tracheal resection. Balloon application should be avoided for the initial 3–4 weeks after surgery.
- Lack of adequate pulmonary reserve to tolerate extended period of airway obstruction

Preoperative Preparation

- Formal direct laryngoscopy and bronchoscopy is required to evaluate stenotic segment and to fully asses the entire airway
- Ensure that all necessary equipment is available and enlist the aid of the corresponding balloon manufacturer's representative if unfamiliar with workings of airway balloon
- Consent should include risk of laryngeal or tracheal rupture along with pneumomediastinum, pneumothorax, and bleeding

Anesthesia Considerations

- Close coordination and communication is needed with an experienced anesthesiologist
- Anesthesiologist should be prepared for oxygen desaturation as the balloon obstructs the airway
- Intravenous steroids are usually administered
- Antibiotics are not required

Equipment Needed

- Rigid endoscope
- A variety of airway balloons

– The author commonly uses the Acclarent Inspira Air Balloon Dilatation System (http://www.acclarent.com/solutions/airway-stenosis/) and the CRETM Pulmonary Balloon Dilator (Boston Scientific, www.boston-scientific.com)
– Balloons come in 5, 7, 10 and 14 mm sizes for the Acclarent system and 8–22 mm for Boston Scientific Pulmonary Balloon Dilator
- Use a balloon size 1 mm larger than the outer diameter of an age-appropriate-sized endotracheal tube. For most children under the age of 2, a 5-mm balloon is appropriate. Children under the age of 13 most likely would benefit from a 7-mm balloon, while most teenagers could use a 10- to 14-mm balloon depending on the size of the airway.
- A balloon inflation device and extension tubing are also required. Specific package inserts describe the recommended pressure settings for each size balloon.

Surgical Procedure

- Ensure equipment is present and prepared prior to patient arriving to the operating room
- Rigid laryngoscopy and bronchoscopy are performed with a 4-mm endoscope in the usual manner. Smaller endoscopes may be used depending on the age of the child and the severity of the stenosis.
- Site of stenosis is identified
- Under endoscopic visualization, the balloon is advanced to the site of the lesion. Half of the balloon is placed distal to the lesion while the other half is placed proximal.
- The balloon is inflated to the specified pressure indicated on the package insert
- The balloon is deflated
- Depending on the desired result, the balloon can be advanced or retracted slightly to ensure a wide area of dilatation. Multiple inflations can be carried out.

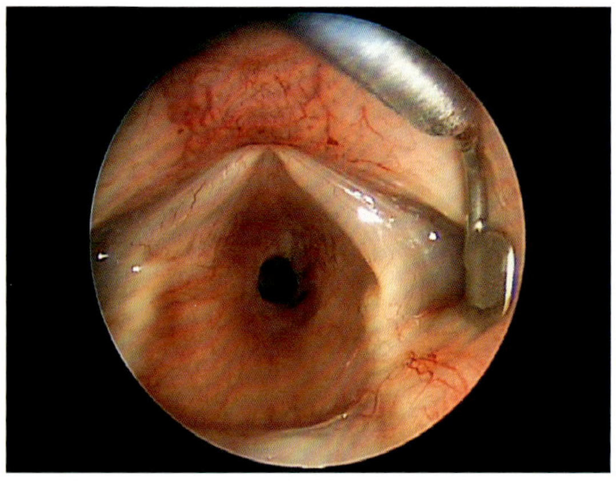

Fig. 1. Preoperative direct laryngoscopy revealed sub-glottic narrowing.

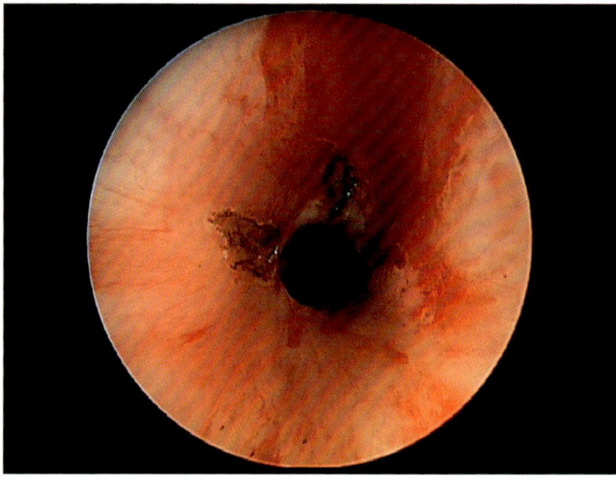

Fig. 2. Using a vocal fold retractor to aid in direct line of site visualization a CO_2 laser was used to make three radial incisions.

Postoperative Care

- Depending on the clinical scenario, the child can be observed or discharged home on the same day
- Frequent dilatations at a rate of every 2 weeks may be necessary

Pearls

- There is no recommended time for balloon inflation. Discussion with providers across the US reveals many options. Some inflate for 10 s, some for 30 s, and some until oxygen desaturation occurs.
- When using the balloons, it may be necessary to employ the provided guide wire in areas of tight stenosis. This may be especially helpful after the balloon is deflated as the guide wire provides rigidity allowing for easier passage.
- Although rare, balloons can be punctured, but it is unlikely that this would cause any harm
- Complication of balloon dilatation can include tracheal rupture, pneumothorax, pneumomediastinitis, and bleeding

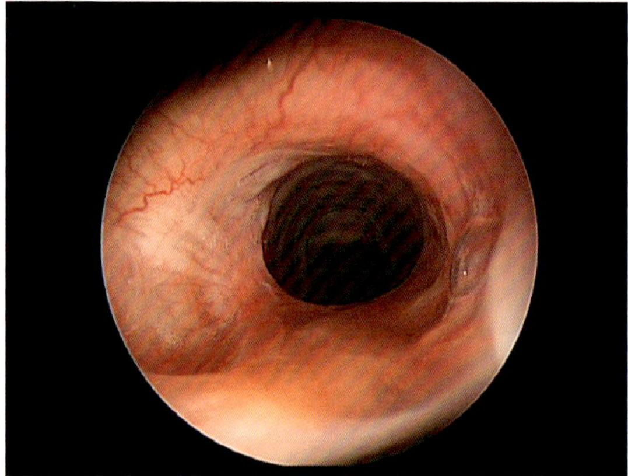

Fig. 3. Two week postoperative pictures revealed a well healed airway and the patient felt that her breathing was easier.

– A minimal amount bleeding is common and does not normally need to be addressed

Case Presentation

A 16-year-old girl with idiopathic subglottic stenosis manifested by shortness of breath with exercise desired a second opinion for management of her airway. She and her family did not desire an open airway procedure, but were amenable to an endoscopic procedure. Her preoperative direct laryngoscopy revealed subglottic narrowing (fig. 1). Using a vocal fold retractor to aid in direct line of site visualization, a CO_2 laser was used to make three radial incisions (fig. 2). After the radial incisions were made, a 14-mm balloon was used to dilate the area (see online suppl. video 1). Two-week postoperative pictures revealed a well-healed airway, and the patient felt that her breathing was easier (fig. 3).

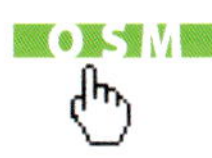

References

1 Bent JP, Shah MB, Nord R, Parikh SR: Balloon dilatation for recurrent stenosis after pediatric laryngotracheoplasty. Ann Otol Rhinol Laryngol 2010;119: 619–627.
2 Durden F, Sobol SE: Balloon laryngoplasty as a primary treatment for subglottic stenosis. Arch Otolaryngol Head Neck Surg 2007;133:772–775.
3 Lee KH, Rutter MJ: Role of balloon dilatation in the management of adult idiopathic subglottic stenosis. Ann Otol Rhinol Laryngol 2008;117:81–84.
4 Ramadan HH: Safety and feasibility of balloon sinuplasty for treatment of chronic rhinosinusistis in children. Ann Otol Rhinol Laryngol 2009;118:161–165.
5 Poe DS, Silvola J, Pyyko I: Balloon dilatation of the cartilaginous Eustachian tube. Otolaryngol Head Neck Surg 2011; 144:563–569.
6 Silver NL, Tassler AB, Malekzadeh S, Harley E: Balloon dilatation for treatment of recurrent choanal atresia. Otolaryngol Head Neck Surg 2008;139:S171.

Christopher J. Hartnick, MD
Professor, Department of Otology and Laryngology
Chief, Division of Pediatric Otolaryngology
Director, Pediatric Airway, Voice and Swallowing Center
Chief Quality Officer
Massachusetts Eye and Ear Infirmary, Harvard Medical School
243 Charles Street
Boston, MA 02116 (USA)
E- Mail christopher_hartnick@meei.harvard.edu

Hartnick CJ, Hansen MC, Gallagher TQ (eds): Pediatric Airway Surgery. Adv Otorhinolaryngol. Basel, Karger, 2012, vol 73, pp 116–122

Endoscopic Posterior Cricoid Split with Rib Grafting

Vikash K. Modi

Pediatric Otolaryngology, Department of Otolaryngology- Head & Neck Surgery, Weill Cornell Medical College, New York, N.Y., USA

Abstract

Bilateral vocal fold immobility(BVFI) can be divided into bilateral vocal fold paralysis and cricoarytenoid joint fixation, which can be accompanied with laryngeal stenosis. In children with BVFI, requiring a tracheostomy, the authors preference, to achieve decannulation, is to perform an endoscopic posterior cricoid split with rib grafting after the age of 1.

Bilateral vocal fold immobility (BVFI) with and without laryngeal stenosis remains a challenging dilemma in the pediatric population. BVFI can be divided into bilateral vocal fold paralysis (BVFP) and cricoarytenoid joint fixation (CAJF), which can be accompanied with posterior glottic stenosis (PGS) and/or subglottic stenosis (SGS). Many children with BVFI resulting in upper airway obstruction will require a tracheostomy.

Etiologies of BVFP are neurological, cardiopulmonary malformations, anoxic injury, trauma, iatrogenic, and idiopathic [1]. The etiology of CAJF, PGS, and SGS are usually related to intubation and subsequent scar formation.

In children with BVFP requiring tracheostomy, there are multiple treatment methods described to allow for decannulation. The goal of surgery is to provide an adequate airway to allow decannulation with minimal impact on speech and swallowing. Vocal cordotomy with/without arytenoidectomy [2], vocal fold suture lateralization, open laryngotracheal reconstruction [3], endoscopic posterior cricoid split with rib grafting [4], and botulinum toxin injection [5], have all been described.

In children with CAJF with and without PGS and/or SGS, numerous treatment options exist to achieve decannulation. Endoscopic procedures include vocal cordotomy, arytenoidectomy, endoscopic mucosal advancement flap, and endoscopic posterior cricoid split with rib grafting. Adjunctive measures include the use of mitomycin C, steroid injection, and botulinum toxin injection. Endoscopic techniques involve the use of cold steel or carbon dioxide laser. Open procedures include scar excision, mucosal grafts/flaps with and without stenting, and laryngotracheal reconstruction.

The decision to perform an endoscopic procedure vs. an open surgery is based on the ability to obtain good endoscopic exposure (see the 'Contraindications' section below). Endoscopic approaches are preferred when possible due to less morbidity resulting in a faster recovery. For example, an EPCG, when compared to an open laryngotracheal reconstruction, does not disrupt the anterior cricoid ring, eliminating the need for stenting. Open procedures should be considered after multiple failures through endoscopic approaches, severe transglottic stenosis, grade 4 SGS, or tracheal stenosis.

When a tracheostomy is present, the author's preference is to perform an EPCG as the first line for an endoscopic approach. This is because it is a nondestructive procedure and has little impact on voice and swallowing. In addition, an EPCG can also address SGS and/or PGS if present. In the author's experience, following an EPCG, there has been no evidence of postoperative aspiration and any dysphonia is temporary. Because an EPCG necessitates a tracheostomy, if no tracheostomy is present, the author's preference is to perform a vocal cordotomy as a first line for an endoscopic approach.

Because more than 50% of BVFP will resolve spontaneously [3, 6], many advocate surgical intervention to achieve decannulation after the child turns one year of age [3].

Indications

- BVFI
- BVFP
- Cricoarytenoid fixation
- With or without laryngeal stenosis
- PGS
- SGS, grade 3 or less

Contraindications

- Poor endoscopic exposure of the larynx
- Retrognathia
- Micrognathia
- Glossoptosis
- Macroglossia
- Retroflexion of the epiglottis
- Severe transglottic stenosis
- Grade 4 SGS
- Tracheal stenosis

Anesthesia Considerations

- FiO_2 at room air
- Laser precautions
- Laser-safe tracheostomy tube (metal)

Preparation

- Direct laryngoscopy and bronchoscopy
- Assess entire airway
- Palpate cricoarytenoid joint
- Laryngeal EMG
- If BVFP, then obtain brain and neck MRI looking for any neurological anomalies
- Special equipment:
- Microscope with laser adapter and micromanipulator
- Carbon dioxide laser
- Lindholm laryngoscope
- Lindholm laryngeal spreader

Procedure

- Preoperative antibiotics
- Patient positioned in supine position with shoulder roll if necessary
- Holinger positioning model (fig. 1; see online suppl. video 1) 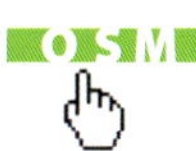
- Lindholm laryngoscope placed in vallecula and suspended from mayo stand
- Lindholm laryngeal spreader inserted in an inverted fashion to retract false vocal folds (see fig. 5b)
- Secured to suspension apparatus with rubber bands (fig. 2)
- Setup operating microscope with CO_2 laser adaptor and micromanipulator
- 5 W and pulse mode
- Straight suction used to protect and push interarytenoid muscles posteriorly to expose posterior cricoid plate

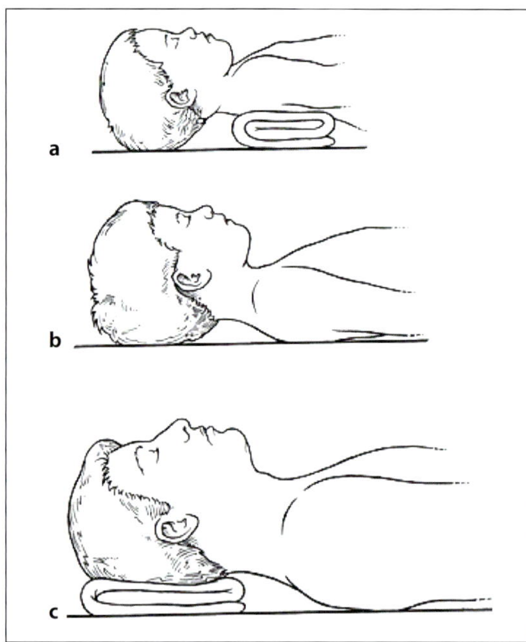

Fig. 1. Proper positioning for laryngoscopy. **a** Premature infants to age 6 or 7. **b** Ages 6–12. **c** Adolescents and adults. Reprinted with kind permission from Holinger L and others: Pediatric Laryngology and Bronchoesophagology, Lippincott-Raven, 1997.

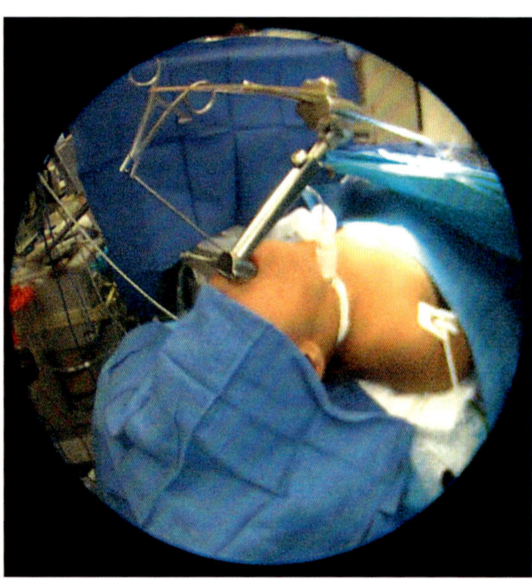

Fig. 2. Setup. Lindholm laryngoscope in suspension, Lindholm spreader fixed to suspension apparatus with rubber bands.

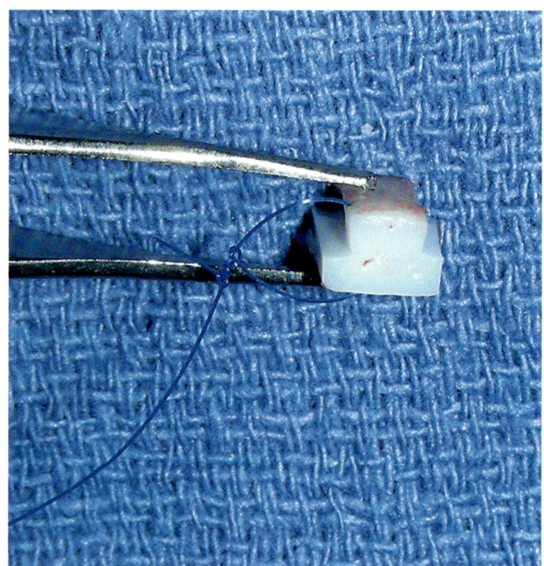

Fig. 3. Rib graft with perichondrium on luminal surface and rescue prolene 5.0 stitch in place.

- Place pressure with straight suction on posterior superior cricoid plate which will rotate the posterior cricoid inferiorly and anteriorly
- Can pull tracheostomy tube anteriorly to help with cricoid rotation
- CO_2 laser used to divide the posterior cricoid plate (see fig. 6, 7)
- Check posterior cricoid intermittently with Hopkins rod telescope (0° and 30°) and a straight suction, curved angle probe or a curved alligator laryngeal forceps
- Do not divide posterior perichondrium
- Do not divide esophageal muscles
- Measure length of posterior cricoid division with a straight suction and measure the width of cricoid distraction with a curved alligator laryngeal forceps
- Harvest 1.5–2.0 cm rib
- Carve rib in T-shaped fashion with perichondrium on the luminal surface (fig. 3)
- Approximately 1 cm in length and 5 mm width of perichondrium

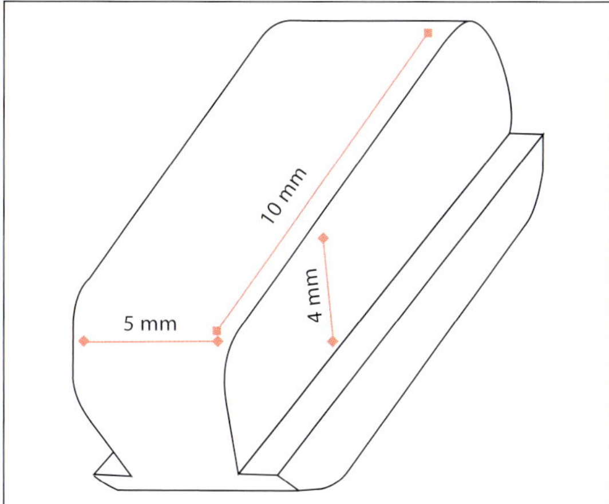

Fig. 4. Average rib graft dimensions.

- 1 mm flanges (fig. 4)
- Place rescue stitch through superior aspect of rib graft with a 5.0 prolene suture on taper needle (fig. 3)
- Remove microscope and use Hopkins rod telescope (0° or 30°)
- Use a stout laryngeal forceps to insert rib graft
- Adjust position of rib graft with curved angle probe
- Cut rescue stitch and pull out
- Remove laryngeal spreader
- Reassess with Hopkins rod telescope

Postoperative Care

- Admission to PICU postoperatively with pulse oximetry
- Do not remove tracheostomy tube
- Humidified oxygen and resume regular diet
- Discharge on postoperative day 3 if tolerating diet and good pain control
- Follow-up laryngoscopy and bronchoscopy at postoperative day 7
- Perform tracheostomy tube change

Pearls

- Proper instruments are essential (Lindholm laryngoscope and laryngeal spreader)
- Put laser on low setting, small spot size, and pulse mode to avoid thermal injury and resorption of cricoid cartilage
- It is important to cut the entire length of the cricoid
- Do not cut through the posterior perichondrium
- Do not undermine perichondrium once through the cricoid
- Important to place prolene rescue stitch when placing graft
- Stitch purpose is to pull the graft out of airway when graft fails to 'seat' in the posterior cricoid split
- Make sure graft is a snug fit with a right angle probe
- If graft does not snap in easily after multiple attempts, then trim graft and repeat
- After completion, reassess with Hopkins rod telescope with and without the laryngeal spreader
- Do not remove tracheostomy tube unless in operating room
- This will safeguard against the possibility of posterior rib graft displacement and aspiration
- Discharge on postoperative day 3
- Plugging of tracheostomy tube with mucous and blood is common and usually occurs 2 days postoperatively

Case Presentation

Case 1
This was a 1.5-year-old child, tracheostomy dependent due to BVFI. Microlaryngoscopy and bronchoscopy revealed CAJF, PGS and grade 2 SGS. Laryngeal EMG revealed good action potentials. Endoscopic posterior cricoid split with rib graft was performed (fig. 5–11).

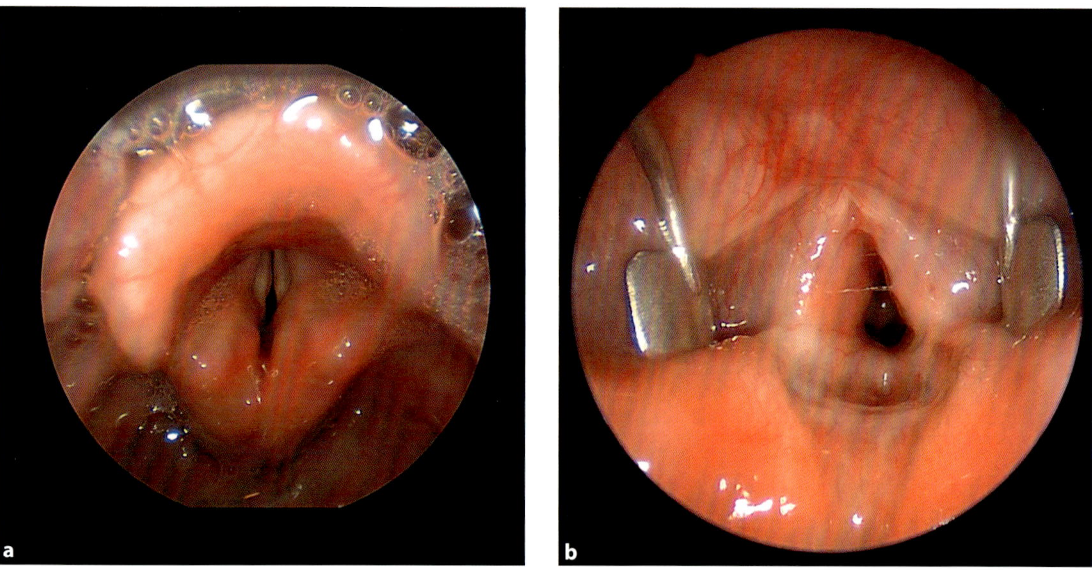

Fig. 5. a. Preoperative view of larynx CAJF and PGS. **b**. Preoperative view of CAJF and PGS with Lindholm laryngeal spreader retracting false vocal folds.

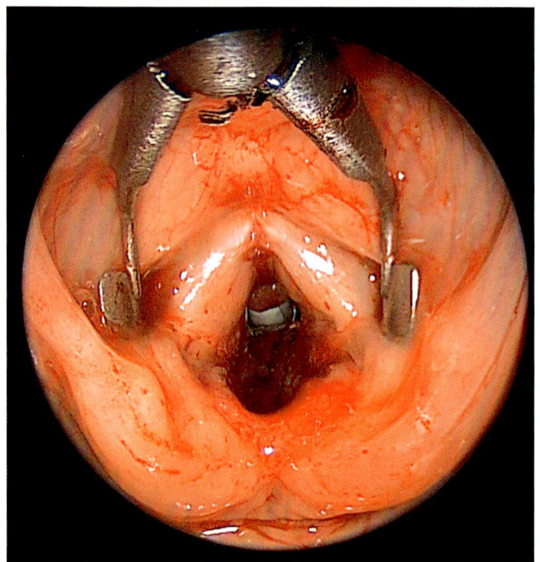

Fig. 6. View after CO_2 laser posterior cricoid split with Lindholm laryngeal spreader retracting false vocal folds. Note that the interarytenoid muscles are left intact.

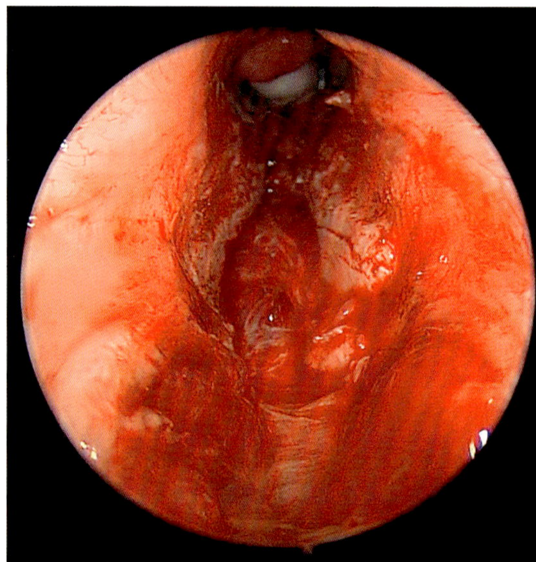

Fig. 7. Zoomed in view of CO_2 laser posterior cricoid split.

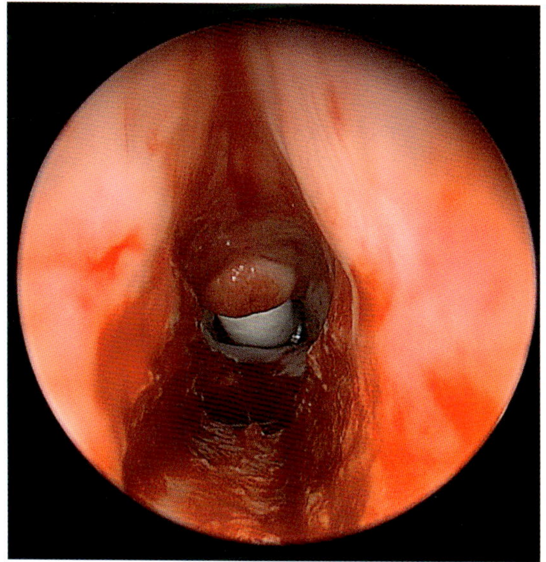

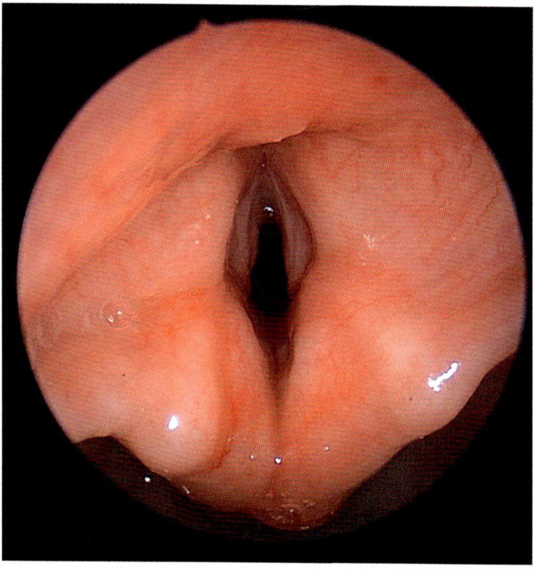

Fig. 8. Zoomed in view of posterior cricoid split with rib graft in place.

Fig. 10. One month after operation.

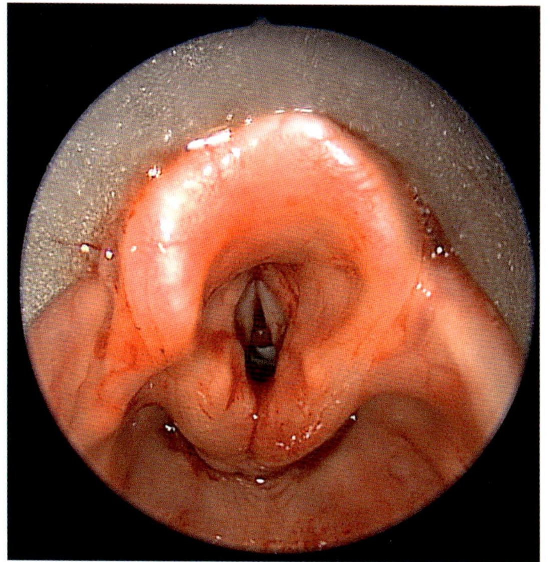

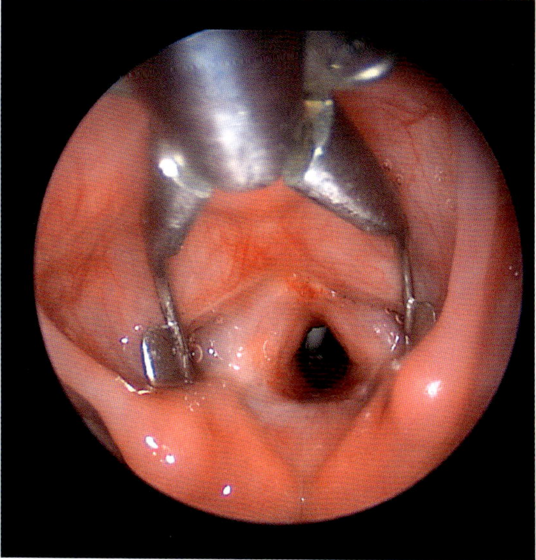

Fig. 9. Immediate postoperative far view without laryngeal spreader.

Fig. 11. Three months after operation with laryngeal spreader.

Case 2

This was a 2-year-old child, tracheostomy dependent due to BVFP. Flexible fiber-optic laryngoscopy at birth revealed no vocal fold motion. An MRI revealed intracranial hemorrhage. At 2 years of age, a flexible fiber-optic laryngoscopy revealed good adduction but poor abduction of the vocal folds. Microlaryngoscopy and bronchoscopy revealed a mobile cricoarytenoid joint and no SGS. Laryngeal EMG revealed sporadic action potentials. Endoscopic posterior cricoid split with rib graft was performed. Patient was decannulated 2 months postoperatively.

References

1 Zbar RI, Smith RJ: Vocal folds paralysis in infants twelve months of age and younger. Otol Head Neck Surg 1996;114:18–21.

2 Aubry K, Leboulanger N, Harris R, Genty E, Denoyelle F, Garabedian EN: Laser arytenoidectomy in the management of bilateral vocal cord paralysis in children. Int J Pediatr Otorhinolarngol 2010;74:451–455.

3 Hartnick CJ, Brigger MT, Wilging JP, Cotton RT, Meyer CM: Surgery for pediatric vocal cord paralysis: a retrospective review. Ann Otol Rhinol Laryngol 2003;112:1–6.

4 Inglis AF, Perkins JA, Manning SC, Mouzakes J: Endoscopic posterior cricoid split and rib grafting in 10 children. Laryngoscope 2003;113:2004–2009.

5 El-Hakim H: Injection of botulinum toxin into external laryngeal muscles in pediatric laryngeal paralysis. Ann Otol Rhinol Laryngol 2008;117:614–620.

6 Cohen Sr, Geller KA, Birns JW, Thompson JW: Laryngeal paralysis in children: a long-term retrospective study. Ann Otol Rhinol Laryngol 1982;91:417–424.

Vikash K. Modi, MD, FAAP
Weill Cornell Medical College
Pediatric Otolaryngology, Department of Otolaryngology- Head & Neck Surgery
428 East 72nd Street, Suite 100
New York, NY 10021 (USA)
E-Mail vkm2001@med.cornell.edu

Hartnick CJ, Hansen MC, Gallagher TQ (eds): Pediatric Airway Surgery. Adv Otorhinolaryngol. Basel, Karger, 2012, vol 73, pp 123–126

Vocal Cordotomy

Vikash K. Modi

Pediatric Otolaryngology, Department of Otolaryngology- Head & Neck Surgery, Weill Cornell Medical College, New York, N.Y., USA

Abstract

Congenital bilateral vocal fold paralysis (BVFP) is the second most common cause of stridor in neonates. Etiologies of BVFP include neurologic, cardiopulmonary malformations, iatrogenic, traumatic, and idiopathic. One half of children with BVFP will require a tracheostomy for upper airway obstruction. Because more than 50% of BVFP will resolve spontaneously, many advocate surgical intervention to achieve decannulation after the age of one. The goal of surgery is to provide an adequate airway to allow decannulation with minimal impact on speech and swallowing. There is no one procedure accepted as the gold standard or first-line treatment to achieve decannulation in children with BVFP. The author's preference is to perform a vocal cordotomy as a first line for an endoscopic approach.

Congenital bilateral vocal fold paralysis (BVFP) is the second most common cause of stridor in neonates [1]. Etiologies of BVFP include neurologic, cardiopulmonary malformations, iatrogenic, traumatic, and idiopathic [2]. One half of children with BVFP will require a tracheostomy for upper airway obstruction [3]. Because more than 50% of BVFP will resolve spontaneously [4], many advocate surgical intervention to achieve decannulation after the age of one [5].

In children with BVFP requiring tracheostomy, multiple treatment methods have been described to achieve decannulation. The goal of surgery is to provide an adequate airway to allow decannulation with minimal impact on speech and swallowing. Vocal cordotomy, vocal cordotomy and arytenoidectomy [6], vocal fold suture lateralization [5], botulinum toxin injection [7], and open [5] vs. endoscopic posterior cricoid split with rib grafting [8] have all been described.

All of these procedures have different effects on speech and swallowing. Each procedure must balance achieving decannulation with the risk of aspiration and a poor voice outcome. The risks and benefits must be assessed and explained to the parents and child in each case. There is no one procedure accepted as the gold standard or first-line treatment to achieve decannulation in children with BVFP.

When a tracheostomy is present, the author's preference is to perform an EPCG as the first line for an endoscopic approach. This is because it is a nondestructive procedure and has little impact on voice and swallowing. In addition, an EPCG can also address subglottic and/or posterior glottic stenosis if present. Because an EPCG necessitates a tracheostomy, if no tracheostomy is present, the author's preference is to perform a vocal cordotomy as a first line for an endoscopic approach.

Indications

- Bilateral vocal fold immobility with upper airway obstruction
- BVFP
- Cricoarytenoid joint fixation

Contraindications

- Children under one year of age
- Due to a high incidence of spontaneous recovery in children with BVFP, many advocate waiting to perform any procedure to achieve decannulation until the child turns one year of age
- Poor endoscopic exposure of the larynx
- Retrognathia
- Micrognathia
- Glossoptosis
- Macroglossia
- Retroflexion of the epiglottis

Anesthesia Considerations

- FiO_2 at room air
- Laser safety precautions
- Laser safe tracheostomy tube (metal) or laser safe endotracheal tube

Preparation

- Laryngeal EMG (see associated chapter for further discussion)
- Consider a cordotomy on side with no action potentials or less activity
- If no action potentials in either vocal fold, MRI of the brain and neck to look for any

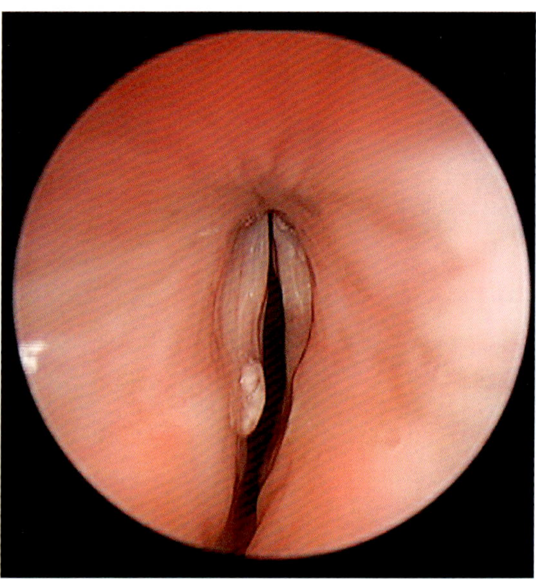

Fig. 1. Preoperative view of larynx without laryngeal spreader.

neurological anomalies as the possible etiology for BVFP
- Special equipment:
- Microscope with laser adapter/micromanipulator
- Carbon dioxide laser
- Lindholm laryngoscope
- Lindholm laryngeal spreader

Procedure

- Preoperative antibiotics
- Patient positioned in supine position with shoulder roll if necessary (see fig. 1 in the chapter 'Endoscopic Posterior Cricoid Split with Rib Grafting', pp. 166–173)
- Lindholm laryngoscope placed in vallecula and suspended from mayo stand
- Lindholm laryngeal spreader placed inverted to retract false vocal folds
- Secured to suspension apparatus with two rubber bands (see fig. 2 in the chapter

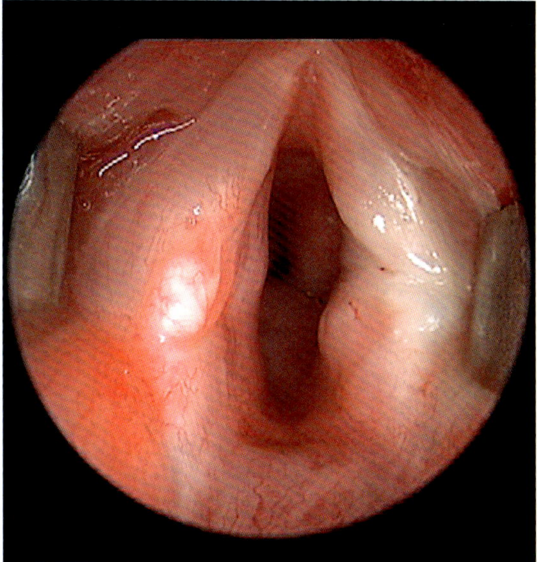

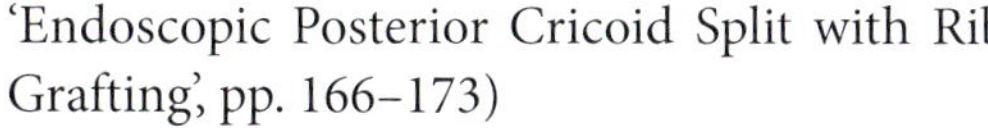

Fig. 2. Preoperative view of larynx with laryngeal spreader.

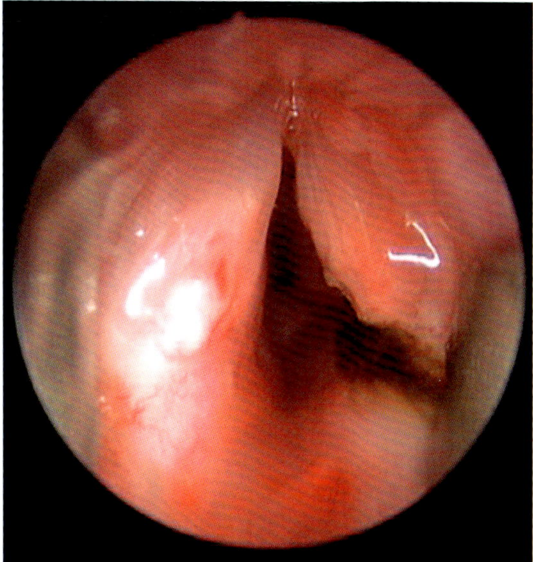

Fig. 3. Postoperative view with laryngeal spreader demonstrating laser cut through entire width of vocal fold.

'Endoscopic Posterior Cricoid Split with Rib Grafting', pp. 166–173)

- Setup operating microscope with CO_2 laser adaptor and micromanipulator
- 5 W and pulse mode
- Carbon dioxide laser used to cut the entire width of the true vocal fold at the level of the vocal process on the desired side (see online suppl. video 1)
- Incision should be carried through the entire length of the conus elasticus to just above the subglottis
- Placement of mitomycin C (0.4 mg/ml) for 3 min is optional

Postoperative Care

- No tracheostomy
- Admission to PICU with continuous pulse oximetry and humidified oxygen
- Tracheostomy
- Admission to floor bed with humidified oxygen

Pearls

- It is important to cut the entire width of the vocal fold and extend the incision through the conus elasticus to avoid rescarring.
- After completion, reassess the laser incision with a Hopkins rod telescope with and without the laryngeal spreader

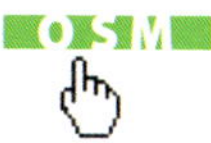

Case Presentation

A newborn presented with biphasic stridor and significant upper airway obstruction resulting in desaturations. The newborn had difficulty with oral intake. Flexible fiberoptic laryngoscopy revealed no vocal fold movement bilaterally. The patient required intubation and underwent a subsequent tracheostomy. MRI revealed a cerebellar infarct. At age one, the patient was still unable to tolerate capping trials, had good adduction but poor abduction of vocal folds. Laryngeal EMG revealed sporadic action potentials bilaterally. Left-sided cordotomy was performed with application of mitomycin C for 3 min (fig. 1–5). The patient progressively tolerated capping trials over the next month. Direct laryngoscopy and bronchoscopy were performed 2–3 months postoperatively, and the patient was admitted for decannulation.

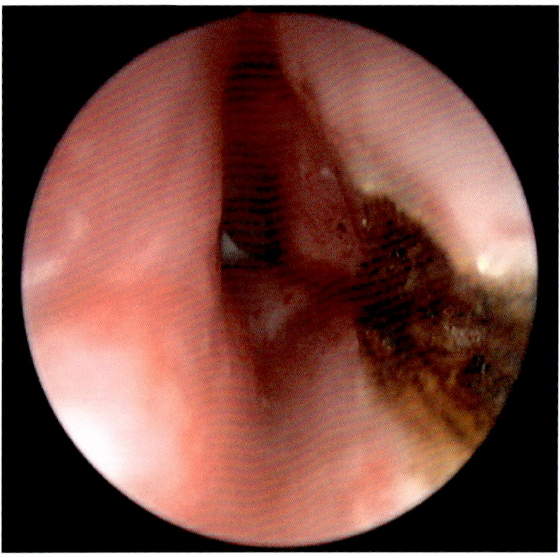

Fig. 4. Postoperative view of larynx zoomed in demonstrating laser cut extending through the conus elasticus.

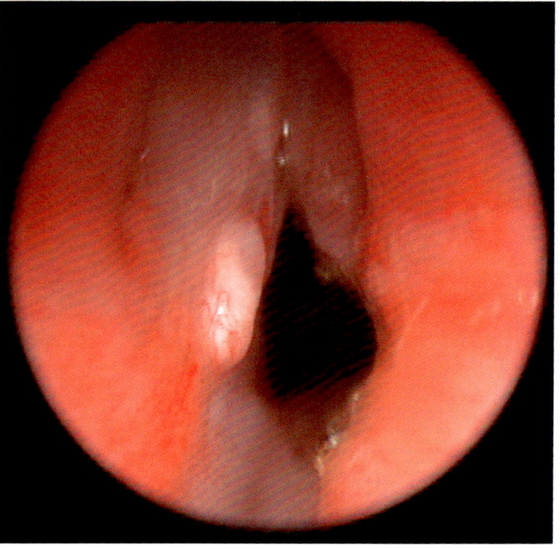

Fig. 5. Postoperative view of larynx without laryngeal spreader.

References

1 Ungkanont K, Friedman EM, Sulek M: A retrospective analysis of airway endoscopy in patients less than 1-month old. Laryngoscope 1998;108:1724–1728.
2 Zbar RI, Smith RJ: Vocal folds paralysis in infants twelve months of age and younger. Otol Head Neck Surg 1996;114:18–21.
3 Dedo DD: Pediatric vocal cord paralysis. Laryngoscope 1979;89:1378–1384.
4 Cohen SR, Geller KA, Birns JW, Thompson JW: Laryngeal paralysis in children: a long-term retrospective study. Ann Otol Rhinol Laryngol 1982;91:417–424.
5 Hartnick CJ, Brigger MT, Wilging JP, Cotton RT, Meyer CM: Surgery for pediatric vocal cord paralysis: a retrospective review. Ann Otol Rhinol Laryngol 2003;112:1–6.
6 Aubry K, Leboulanger N, Harris R, Genty E, Denoyelle F, Garabedian EN: Laser arytenoidectomy in the management of bilateral vocal cord paralysis in children. Int J Pediatr Otorhinolaryngol 2010;74:451–455.
7 El-Hakim H: Injection of botulinum toxin into external laryngeal muscles in pediatric laryngeal paralysis. Ann Otol Rhinol Laryngol 2008;117:614–620.
8 Inglis AF, Perkins JA, Manning SC, Mouzakes J: Endoscopic posterior cricoid split and rib grafting in 10 children. Laryngoscope 2003;113:2004–2009.

Vikash K. Modi, MD, FAAP
Weill Cornell Medical College
Pediatric Otolaryngology, Department of Otolaryngology- Head & Neck Surgery
428 East 72nd Street, Suite 100
New York, NY 10021 (USA)
E-Mail vkm2001@med.cornell.edu

Hartnick CJ, Hansen MC, Gallagher TQ (eds): Pediatric Airway Surgery. Adv Otorhinolaryngol. Basel, Karger, 2012, vol 73, pp 127–131

Endoscopic Choanal Atresia Repair

Thomas Q. Gallagher[a] · Christopher J. Hartnick[b]

[a]LCDR, MC, USN, Department of Otolaryngology, Naval Medical Center Portsmouth, Portsmouth, Va., and [b]Department of Otology and Laryngology, Massachusetts Eye & Ear Infirmary, Boston, Mass., USA

Abstract

Congenital choanal atresia (CA) is relatively rare, with an incidence of 1 in 7,000 births with a majority being the mixed bony-membranous type. There are 5 described methods of CA repair: transpalatal, transnasal, sublabial-transnasal, transantral, and transseptal approaches. Transpalatal and transnasal have been the most popular in the last several decades with transnasal becoming the preferred technique with the advent of endoscopic instruments and techniques. In this chapter, the authors seek to describe their techniques for endoscopic transnasal repair of CA including surgical pearls for success.

Congenital choanal atresia (CA) is relatively rare with an incidence of 1 in 7,000 births [1]. Analysis of CA by computed tomography (CT) reveals 70% are mixed bony-membranous and 30% are bony [2]. Neonates are obligate nasal breathers making bilateral CA a medically urgent diagnosis. However, workup for associated congenital anomalies is necessary prior to surgical repair.

A recent retrospective case series of 129 children found CA to be an isolated finding in 26.4% of the cohort and associated with other anomalies 73.6% of the time [3]. CHARGE (coloboma, heart defect, atresia choanae, retarded growth, genitourinary defects, and ear abnormalities) syndrome was the most common diagnosis (25.6%) identified in their cohort. The ratio of unilateral to bilateral CA is about 1:1 with unilateral cases more likely to be isolated and bilateral cases more likely to be associated with specific disorders or multiple congenital anomalies.

Teratogenicity is another possible etiology of CA. Some recent reports and case series in the literature have demonstrated unilateral and bilateral CA in mothers treated for hyperthyroidism during pregnancy with methimazole [4, 5].

There are 5 described methods of CA repair: transpalatal, transnasal, sublabial-transnasal, transantral, and transseptal approaches. Transpalatal and transnasal have been the most popular in the last several decades with transnasal becoming the preferred technique with the advent of endoscopic instruments and techniques.

Bilateral CA is an urgent diagnosis and requires surgical treatment. Unilateral CA may be observed to allow time for the infant to feed and grow prior to surgical repair unless there is difficulty with breathing, feeding, or weight gain.

Indications

- Bilateral congenital CA
- Unilateral CA
- Feeding/weight gain difficulties
- Breathing difficulties
- Unilateral rhinorrhea/nasal dyspnea as a child or adolescent

Contraindications

- Skull base anatomic anomalies
- Anterior nasal obstruction limiting passage of endoscopes through the nose
- Pyriform aperture stenosis
- CHARGE syndrome
- Asher et al. [6] advocated delaying CA repair until 2 years of age and performing a tracheotomy instead in children with CHARGE due to the high risk of airway complications in their cohort

Anesthesia Considerations

None.

Preparation

- CT scan evaluation looking at bony and membranous components as well as adjacent anatomy
- Sagittal reconstruction is helpful in evaluation for skull base anomalies
- Oxymetazoline-soaked pledgets to decongest nares

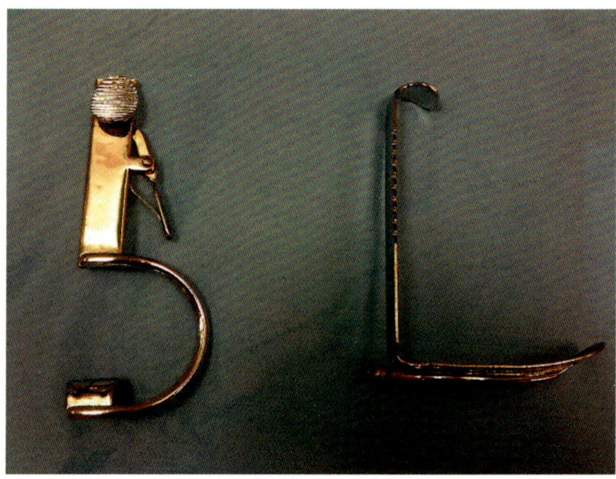

Fig. 1. Infant mouth gag.

- Special equipment:
- Hegar urethral sounds
- Karl Storz (Tuttlingen, Germany) 120° degree endoscope with uvula/soft palate retractor
- Medtronic (Minneapolis, Minn., USA) 2.9-mm Silver Bullet rotatable shaver
- Medtronic 4-mm CA diamond burr

Procedure

- Patient positioned in modified Rose position with a Crow-Davis mouth gag suspended off the mayo stand
- We utilize a custom infant mouth gag for these cases (fig. 1)
- A red rubber catheter is utilized in the unilateral cases to assist with retracting the palate. In a bilateral case, this can be inserted after the atretic membrane has been taken down.
- Urethral sounds are used to serially dilate the atresia under direct vision using 120° endoscope (fig. 2)
- The Medtronic Silver Bullet shaver is used to remove the membranous atresia (fig. 3; online suppl. video 1)
- A pediatric sinus backbiter is used to take down portions of the boney atresia as well as

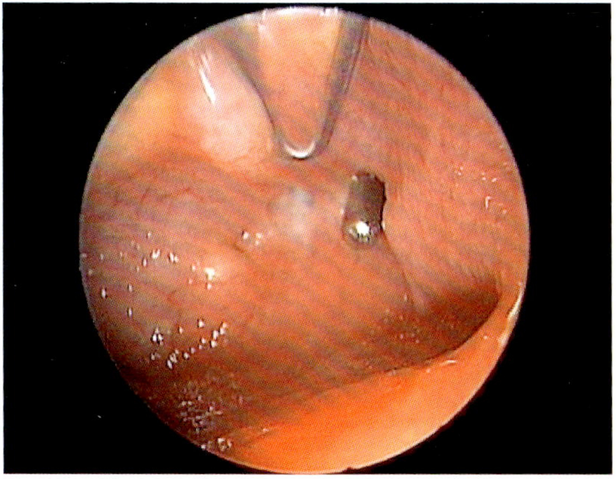

Fig. 2. Urethral sound dilating the left choanae under direct vision in a patient with bilateral choanal atresia.

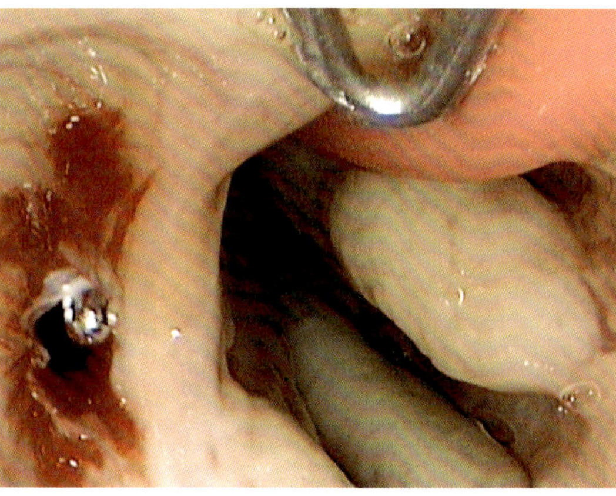

Fig. 3. Silver Bullet microdebrider removing membranous atresia in a patient with unilateral right sided choanal atresia.

the posterior vomer in order to enlarge the posterior nasopharynx (fig. 4)

– Utilization of the contralateral nasal passageway is helpful to remove all the necessary tissue

• A combination of the Silver Bullet blade, diamond burr and backbiter are used to create a large common posterior cavity. Care is taken to avoid skull base and sphenopalatine foramen.

– Medial and inferior dissection is safe

Postoperative Care

• Nasal saline spray is used several times daily with bulb suction for clearance of clot and crusting

• Stents are only utilized in this procedure for neonates with bilateral CA

– Customized endotracheal tubes of the appropriate size are placed to prevent immediate postoperative obstruction

– Removed at 2 weeks

• Repeat endoscopy in 2–3 weeks in the operating room with debridement as necessary

Fig. 4. A backbiter passed through the opening created by the microdebrider is taking down the vomer to create a large posterior 'common cavity' in a patient with unilateral right sided choanal atresia.

Pearls

• It is important to directly observe the dilation of the atresia with the urethral sounds

• A sufficient amount of posterior vomer is to be removed in order to avoid restenosis

• Utilization of the contralateral nasal passageway for exposure and passage of instruments is essential

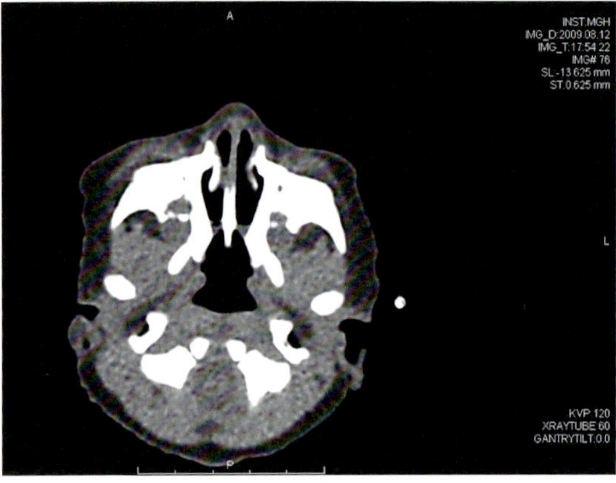

Fig. 5. Preoperative CT.

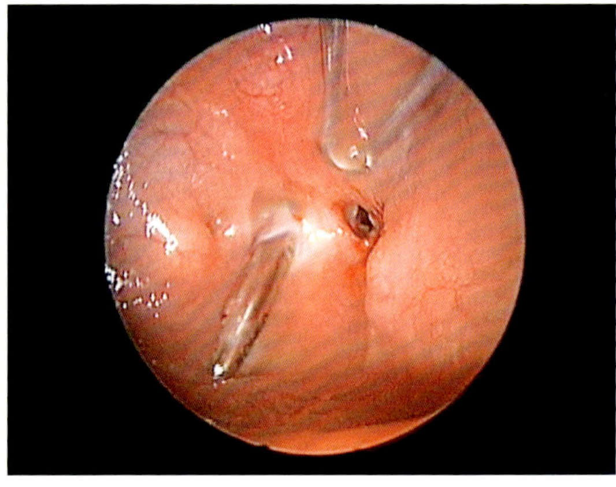

Fig. 7. Silver Bullet shaver utilized during repair.

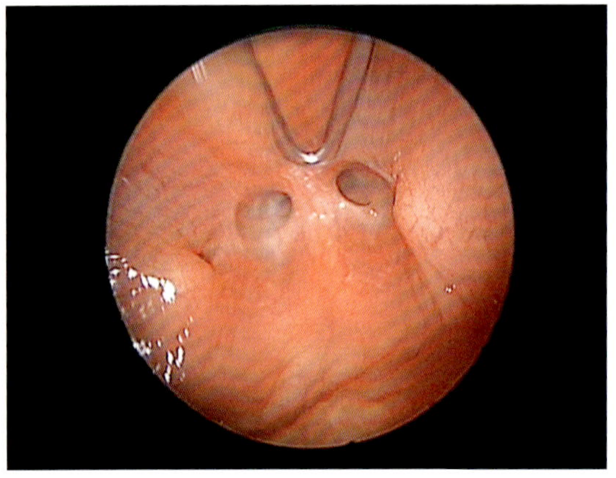

Fig. 6. Preoperative endoscopy using the 120° scope demonstrating bilateral atresia.

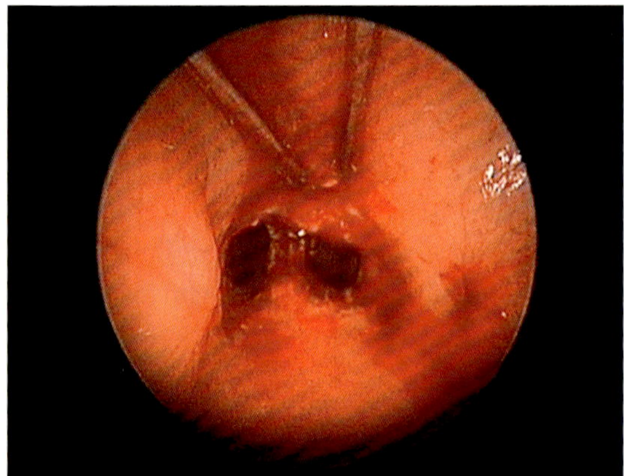

Fig. 8. Postoperative view.

Case Presentation

A 6-day-old female presented with respiratory distress, cyanosis with feeding and poor PO intake. A CT scan of the maxillofacial region was performed (fig. 5) and revealed mixed bony-membranous bilateral atresia. Endoscopic atresia repair and preoperative endoscopy (fig. 6) were performed. Urethral sounds were used to dilate choanae. Microdebrider Silver Bullet was used to enlarge membranous atresia (fig. 7), and Backbiter and diamond atresia burr to enlarge the common cavity. The postoperative view is shown in figure 8. No stents were placed; patient used saline rinses for 2 weeks. Follow-up endoscopy in clinic showed patent choanae with symptomatic improvement.

References

1 Carpenter RJ, Neel HB: Correction of congenital choanal atresia in children and adults. Laryngoscope 1977;87:1304–1311.
2 Brown OE, Pownell P, Manning SC: Choanal atresia: a new anatomic classification and clinical management applications. Laryngoscope 1996;106:97–101.
3 Burrow AT, Saal HM, de Alarcon A, Martin LJ, Cotton RT, et al: Characterization of congenital anomalies in individuals with choanal atresia. Arch Otolaryngol Head Neck Surg 2009;135:543–547.
4 Barbero P, Valdez R, Rodriguez, et al: Choanal atresia associated with maternal hyperthyroidism treated with methimazole: a case-control study. Am J Med Genet A 2008;146A:2390–2395.
5 Clementi M, Gianantonio E, Cassina M, Leoncini E, et al: Treatment of hyperthyroidism in pregnancy and birth defects. J Clin Endocrinol Metab 2010;95:E337–E341.
6 Asher BF, McGill TJ, Kaplan L, Friedman EM, Healy GB: Airway complications in CHARGE association. Arch Otolaryngol Head Neck Surg 1990;116:594–595.

Christopher J. Hartnick, MD
Professor, Department of Otology and Laryngology
Chief, Division of Pediatric Otolaryngology
Director, Pediatric Airway, Voice and Swallowing Center
Chief Quality Officer
Massachusetts Eye and Ear Infirmary, Harvard Medical School
243 Charles Street
Boston, MA 02116 (USA)
E-Mail christopher_hartnick@meei.harvard.edu

Hartnick CJ, Hansen MC, Gallagher TQ (eds): Pediatric Airway Surgery. Adv Otorhinolaryngol. Basel, Karger, 2012, vol 73, pp 132–136

Endoscopic Resection of Juvenile Nasopharyngeal Angiofibroma

Derek J. Rogers · Scott E. Bevans · Wayne J. Harsha

Otolaryngology-Head and Neck Surgery, Madigan Army Medical Center, Tacoma, Wash., USA

Abstract

Juvenile nasopharyngeal angiofibromas remain rare tumors representing approximately 0.05% of head and neck tumors. The typical presentation is a male teenager with recurrent epistaxis and nasal obstruction. These tumors were traditionally approached via external and/or intraoral incisions, but many are amenable to endoscopic removal. Preoperative embolization of major feeding vessels to these tumors by interventional radiology has resulted in significantly less blood loss and facilitated endoscopic resection. The following chapter discusses endoscopic resection of juvenile nasopharyngeal angiofibromas and outlines pertinent anatomy while covering important surgical techniques. Appropriate patient selection, anesthesia considerations, surgical preparation and techniques, and postoperative care are discussed. A case presentation is included with preoperative imaging and an accompanying video to demonstrate these surgical techniques.

Juvenile nasopharyngeal angiofibromas (JNAs) remain rare tumors representing approximately

The views expressed in this article are those of the authors and do not necessarily reflect the official policy or position of the Department of the Army, Department of Defense, or the United States Government.

Derek J. Rogers, Scott E. Bevans, and Wayne J. Harsha are military service members. This work was prepared as part of their official duties. Title 17 .S.C. 105 provides that 'Copyright protection under this title is not available for any work of the United States Government.' Title 17 U.S.C. 101 defines a United States Government work as a work prepared by a military service member or employee of the United States Government as part of that person's official duties.

0.05% of head and neck tumors [1]. The typical presentation is a male teenager with recurrent epistaxis and nasal obstruction. Patients are frequently treated for allergies initially before being referred to an otolaryngologist. The epistaxis can be quite severe, even requiring a transfusion.

These tumors were traditionally approached via external (lateral rhinotomy, midfacial degloving, infratemporal) and/or intraoral incisions (transmaxillary or transpalatal), but many are amenable to endoscopic removal. When compared to the traditional approaches, the endoscopic approach leads to less intraoperative blood loss, fewer complications, lower rate of recurrence, and shorter hospital stay [2]. Preoperative embolization of major feeding vessels to these tumors by interventional radiology has resulted in significantly less blood loss and facilitated endoscopic resection [3]. Since these tumors originate from the sphenopalatine artery, the endoscopic approach focuses on gaining access to the sphenopalatine foramen, while ensuring the entire tumor is freed from surrounding structures.

The following chapter discusses endoscopic resection of JNAs and outlines pertinent anatomy while covering important surgical techniques. Appropriate patient selection, anesthesia considerations, surgical preparation and techniques, and postoperative care are discussed. A case presentation is included with preoperative imaging and an accompanying video to demonstrate these surgical techniques.

Relevant Anatomy

- Sphenopalatine artery is a terminal branch of internal maxillary artery, which is a branch of external carotid artery
- Sphenopalatine foramen is located along the lateral nasal wall immediately posterior to the crista ethmoidalis, opening into the middle and superior meatus
- Most individuals have two or more branches from the sphenopalatine artery

Indications

- Tumor limited to nose or nasopharynx
- Tumor extending into paranasal sinuses or pterygopalatine fossa
- Tumor with medial infratemporal fossa involvement
- Some tumors with limited intracranial extension (extradural in parasellar region)
- To facilitate combined or open approaches

Contraindications

- Tumor with lateral infratemporal fossa involvement
- Tumor with extensive parasellar extension or surrounding optic nerve
- Tumor with intradural involvement
- Tumor with cavernous sinus involvement

Anesthesia Considerations

- Hypotensive general anesthesia

- Patient lies supine in reverse Trendelenburg position
- Oral RAE® endotracheal tube
- Obtain 2 units of autologous blood banked the week before surgery

Preparation

- Preoperative:
- CT scan of the paranasal sinuses with and without contrast to evaluate for bony erosion
- MRI of the paranasal sinuses with and without contrast to evaluate soft tissue extent of tumor including neural foramina and intracranial involvement
- Angiogram for embolization of major feeding vessels to the tumor 24–72 h before surgery
- Intraoperative:
- Surgeon should consider sitting or bracing his/her arm holding the endoscope
- Strongly consider intraoperative image guidance CT
- Use an endoscope with an automatic cleaner such as Endo-Scrub®
- Have suction bipolar electrocautery, suction Freer elevator, suction Blakesley or Kerrison forceps, and hemoclip applier available
- Greater palatine foramina are injected with lidocaine with epinephrine intraorally
- Septum, uncinate process, and root of the middle turbinate on side of tumor are injected with lidocaine with epinephrine
- Both nasal cavities are packed for 10 min with cottonoid pledgets soaked in oxymetazoline

Procedure

- Remove pledgets from nasal cavities [4]
- Visualize nasal cavity containing the tumor with endoscope
- Amputate the inferior aspect of the middle turbinate with scissors (fig. 1)

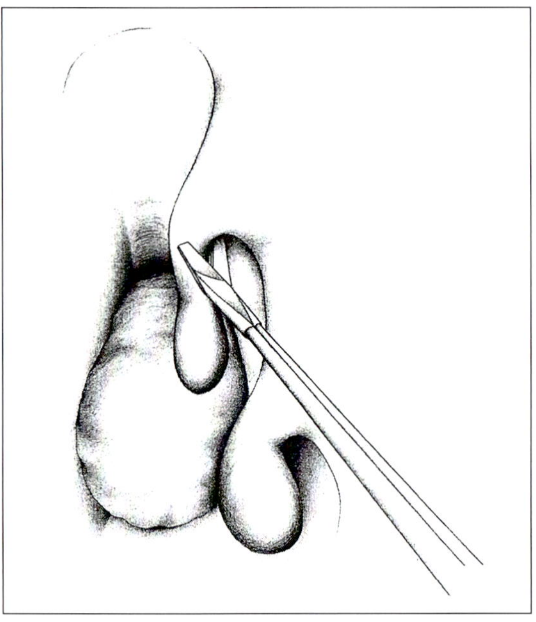

Fig. 1. Inferior aspect of middle turbinate is amputated with scissors. Reprinted from Wormald and Van Hasselt [4] by permission of SAGE Publications.

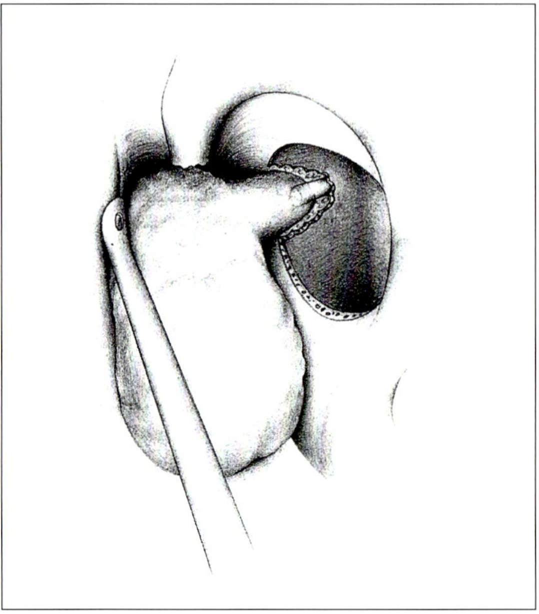

Fig. 2. Sphenopalatine artery and tumor pedicle are exposed by removing posterior wall of maxillary sinus. Reprinted from Wormald and Van Hasselt [4] by permission of SAGE Publications.

- Perform uncinectomy and wide middle meatal antrostomy
- Enlarge middle meatal antrostomy until the posterior wall of the maxillary sinus is visualized
- Consider posterior septectomy to allow better visualization and access from opposite nasal cavity
- Perform anterior and posterior ethmoidectomy until sphenoid rostrum is identified
- Perform sphenoidotomy to ensure tumor does not extend into sphenoid
- Expose the sphenopalatine artery and tumor pedicle by removing the posterior wall of the maxillary sinus (fig. 2). Tumor may extend beyond pterygopalatine fossa into infratemporal fossa.
- Dissect tumor off of surrounding structures using suction Freer elevator
- Tumor is frequently adherent to septum, sphenoid rostrum, skull base and nasopharynx; use suction bipolar cautery to ablate feeding vessels along tumor surface and sharply dissect tumor free with suction Freer, scalpel, or sickle knife.
- Work the entire tumor free until all that remains is its pedicle
- Apply hemoclips to sphenopalatine artery, ligate pedicle with endoscopic bipolar cautery and scissors, and deliver tumor through nasopharynx and mouth. Note: some surgeons ligate the sphenopalatine artery before dissecting the tumor free from surrounding structures.
- Inspect entire mucosal area that involved tumor and send biopsies to clear margins
- Obtain hemostasis with endoscopic bipolar cautery
- Apply hemostatic sinus dressing, such as Arista^{TM} powder or Stammberger Sinu-foam^{TM}
- See online supplementary video 1 for demonstration of the aforementioned steps for a JNA originating off of the right sphenopalatine artery

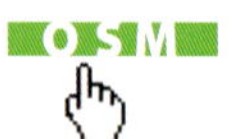

Postoperative Care

- Consider admitting patient for overnight observation
- If intraoperative blood loss was significant, consider blood transfusion
- Oxymetazoline is used as needed for epistaxis
- Start nasal saline irrigations at least twice a day on first postoperative day
- Analgesia with oxycodone or hydrocodone
- Instruct patient not to blow his/her nose
- First postoperative visit within one week

Pearls

- Preoperative embolization of tumor by interventional radiology is paramount
- Intraoperative navigation is extremely helpful
- Dissection is facilitated by suction bipolar electrocautery, suction Freer elevator, suction Blakesley or Kerrison forceps, and hemoclip applier
- If tumor involves lateral infratemporal fossa or parasellar region, be prepared for open approach as well

Case Presentation

A 16-year-old otherwise healthy male presented with progressively worsening nasal obstruction and recurrent epistaxis. The epistaxis had become more frequent and severe. The patient was treated with nasal steroids and antihistamines with no improvement in symptoms. His physical exam revealed a large vascular mass filling his right posterior nasal cavity and nasopharynx (fig. 3). A CT (fig. 4) and MRI (fig. 5) were obtained and confirmed the presence of a right enhancing sinonasal tumor extending from the sphenopalatine foramen with only medial infratemporal fossa involvement. Angiogram with embolization was performed on the tumor one day before surgery. The patient underwent endoscopic resection of the tumor and was admitted for 24-hour observation. His postoperative course was uneventful, and nasal endoscopy revealed no evidence of tumor.

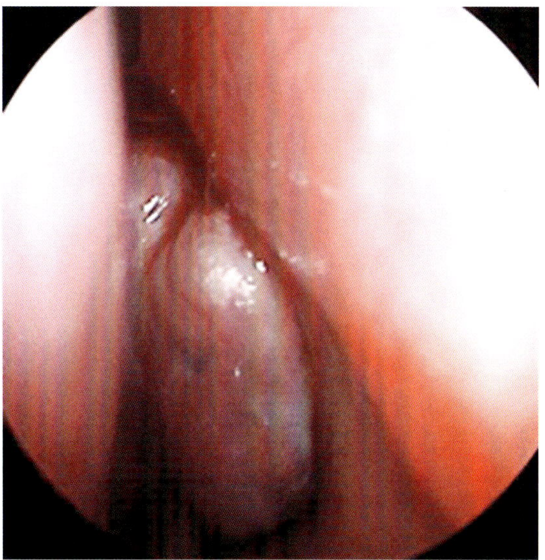

Fig. 3. Large vascular mass filling right nasal cavity.

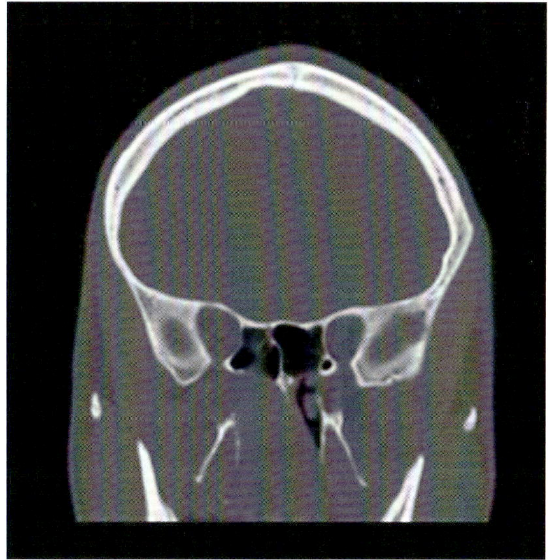

Fig. 4. Soft tissue mass causing enlargement of right sphenopalatine foramen.

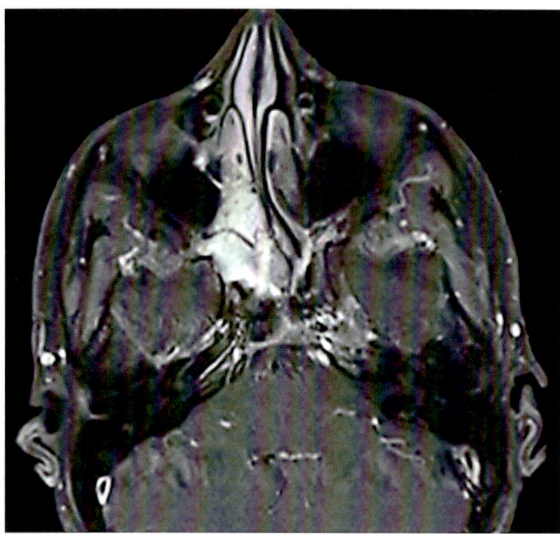

Fig. 5. MRI with contrast confirms a vascular mass involving only medial aspect of right infratemporal fossa.

References

1 Herman P, Lot G, Chapot R, et al: Long-term follow-up of juvenile nasapharyngeal angiofibromas: analysis of recurrences. Laryngoscope 1999;109:140–147.

2 Pryor SG: Endoscopic versus traditional approaches for excision of juvenile nasopharyngeal angiofibroma. Laryngoscope 2005;115:1201–1207.

3 Schroth G, Haldermann AR, Mariani L, et al: Preoperative embolization of paragangliomas and angiofibromas. Arch Otolaryngol Head Neck Surg 1996;122:1320–1325.

4 Wormald PJ, Van Hasselt: Endoscopic removal of juvenile angiofibromas. Otolaryngol Head Neck Surg 2003;129:684–691.

Derek J. Rogers, MD
Madigan Army Medical Center
Otolaryngology-Head and Neck Surgery
9040A Fitzsimmons Dr.
Tacoma, WA 98431 (USA)
E-Mail derek.john.rogers@us.army.mil

Hartnick CJ, Hansen MC, Gallagher TQ (eds): Pediatric Airway Surgery. Adv Otorhinolaryngol. Basel, Karger, 2012, vol 73, pp 137–144

Surgery for Velopharyngeal Insufficiency

Gregory Capra · Matthew T. Brigger

Department of Otolaryngology, Head and Neck Surgery, Naval Medical Center San Diego, San Diego, Calif., USA

Abstract

Velopharyngeal inadequacy may be learned, neurologic, or anatomic in origin. Velopharyngeal insufficiency specifically refers to an anatomic deficiency, which subsequently impairs resonant control of speech and intraoral pressure for orally directed speech sounds. Preoperative speech therapy is useful, and in some children may provide definitive treatment. However, surgery is the foundation of effective treatment in most patients with anatomic defects and, when used appropriately, has been shown to result in resolution of velopharyngeal insufficiency in 62–98% of cases. In this chapter, the authors review velopharyngeal inadequacy and discuss the techniques necessary for successful surgical treatment.

Velopharyngeal inadequacy may be learned, neurologic, or anatomic in origin. Velopharyngeal insufficiency (VPI) specifically refers to insufficient tissue closure due to an anatomic deficiency, which subsequently impairs resonant control of speech and intra-oral pressure for orally directed speech sounds [1, 2]. Many cases are syndromic

in nature and due to abnormal craniofacial development with cleft palate anomalies being the most common cause. Other notable etiologies include velo-cardio-facial syndrome (chromosomal microdeletion of 22q11.2), neuromuscular disorders, tonsillar hypertrophy and iatrogenic causes such as post-adenoidectomy VPI [3–5]. Airflow through the nasopharynx is determined by the sphincter action of the velopharyngeal port, which is derived from the superior pharyngeal constrictor and the five muscles that constitute the soft palate. The palatal muscles act to elevate, tense, and approximate the soft palate to the posterior pharyngeal wall, while the superior constrictor medializes the nasopharyngeal wall to close the velopharyngeal port [6–9]. The resultant four velopharyngeal closure patterns are coronal, circular, circular with Passavant's ridge, and sagittal (fig. 1) [10].

All children with VPI should be evaluated by a speech and language pathologist. Preoperative speech therapy is useful, and in some children may provide definitive treatment [11–13]. However, in most children the defect is anatomic in nature and requires correction of the anatomic defect. Obturators and palatal lifts may benefit patients when surgery is contraindicated, wide clefts are present, or neuromuscular deficits of the soft palate exist [14]. However, surgery is the foundation of effective treatment in patients with anatomic defects and, when used appropriately, has been

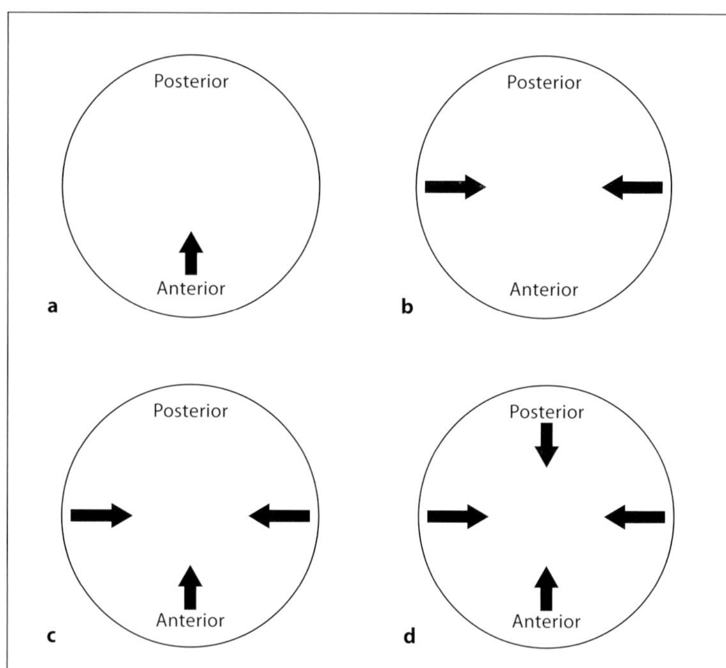

Fig.1. Pharyngeal closure patterns important in VPI. **a** Coronal. **b** Sagittal. **c** Circular. **d** Circular with the Passavant ridge. Reprinted with kind permission from WebMD.com.

shown to result in resolution of VPI in 62–98% of cases [15–24].

Selection of an appropriate surgical procedure is predicated upon the preoperative anatomy and velopharyngeal closure pattern. Further considerations include other comorbidities including the presence of sleep-disordered breathing or aberrant anatomy.

Preoperative Evaluation

- All children with VPI where surgical intervention is considered require detailed evaluation of velopharyngeal anatomy. Flexible nasendoscopy during volitional vocalizing tasks has proved invaluable in diagnosis and surgical planning. It is best suited for children 6 years or older because they can better cooperate; however, it can be used successfully in younger children. Multiview fluoroscopy is an alternative that is widely used to provide accurate description of velopharyngeal closure patters.
- Evaluation by a speech and language pathologist is critical to confirm the diagnosis and potentially identify associated functional speech abnormalities. Speech therapy may be useful to establish accurate speech patterns to optimize surgical success.
- Objective measures of hypernasality such as nasometry or weighted speech scales may prove useful in diagnosis, postoperative therapy, and evaluating outcomes
- Screening for carotid artery medialization with contrast-enhanced CT scan or magnetic resonance angiography is recommended in patients suspected to have velo-cardio-facial syndrome
- Careful consideration of the role of the palatine tonsils in speech is individualized for each child. Evaluation of sleep-disordered breathing symptoms is important to identify

at risk children preoperatively. Removal of hypertrophic tonsils may be useful to prevent or treat postoperative OSA. In some children, hypertrophic tonsils may contribute to velopharyngeal closure. Conversely, some children may experience VPI secondary to hypertrophic tonsils preventing adequate palatal movement. Tonsillectomy is generally performed 6 weeks prior to primary velopharyngeal surgery, but has been described as a concurrent procedure.

Superior-Based Pharyngeal Flap

Indications
- Goal is to effectively obturate the velopharynx using a posterior pharyngeal wall myomucosal flap that provides a central bulk of tissue, while allowing airflow through lateral ports
- VPI associated with sagittal closure patterns are most amenable to pharyngeal flaps as the lateral wall motion is used to control the release of air through the ports

Contraindications
Special consideration must be made in children with sleep-disordered breathing as postoperative obstructive sleep apnea is a reported complication.

Anesthesia Considerations
- General endotracheal anesthesia is required
- A high level of suspicion should be maintained for velo-cardio-facial syndrome and coexistent cardiac abnormalities

Preparation
- Preoperative:
- Review nasendoscopy or multiview fluoroscopy
- Intraoperative:
- Shoulder roll as necessary for neck extension

- Insert Dingman mouth gag and place into Rose position
- Posterior nasopharyngeal wall is evaluated and palpated to identify anomalous vasculature
- The senior author routinely administers perioperative antibiotics

Procedure
For details of the procedure, see figure 2 and on-line supplementary video 1. 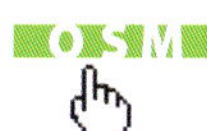
- Flap width is estimated to be the distance of the posterior tonsillar pillars. The inferior extent is approximately equivalent to the midpoint of the tonsillar fossa. An estimate of flap length can be made by measuring the distance of the free edge of the soft palate to the posterior pharyngeal wall.
- Proposed pharyngeal incision lines are injected with 1% lidocaine with 1:100,000 epinephrine to aid in hemostasis and hydrodissection of the surgical plane
- The nasal aspect of the soft palate is injected with the same lidocaine-epinephrine solution
- A superiorly based pharyngeal flap is elevated by incising down to the level of the prevertebral fascia. The proper plane is devoid of major vessels. Monopolar cautery may be used as needed to achieve hemostasis.
- A slight lateral curve at the superior aspect of the lateral incisions may be helpful to create the lateral ports
- Elevation proceeds from an inferior point superiorly high into the nasopharynx to the level of natural velopharyngeal closure and can be correlated with landmarks seen on preoperative nasendoscopy
- A horizontal incision is made on the nasal surface of the soft palate. The soft palate may be split in the midline to facilitate visualization.
- Sizing of the lateral ports is done with a 3.5 endotracheal tube in children and maintained in position during inset of the flap

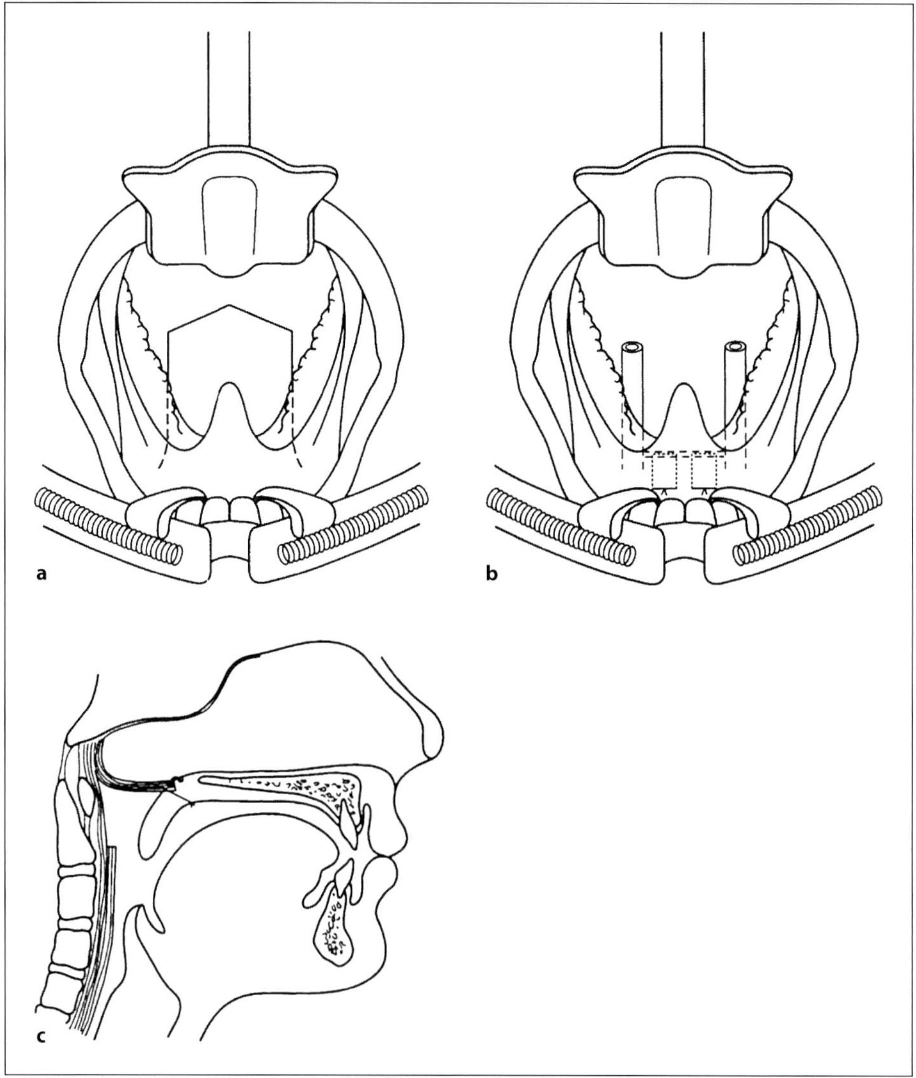

Fig. 2. **a** Superiorly based posterior pharyngeal flap pharyngeal wall incisions. Inferior edge of flap will be inset into nasal surface of the soft palate. **b** Flap inset into position with endotracheal tubes in place creating lateral ports. **c** Sagittal view of flap in position. Reprinted with kind permission from Bluestone CD & Rosenfeld RM, Surgical Atlas of Pediatric Otolaryngology, 2002, BC Decker.

- 4-0 vicryl sutures are used to sew the superiorly based flap to the nasal surface of the soft palate
- 3-0 vicryl sutures are placed in a horizontal mattress fashion through the soft palate and flap on either side of the midline. This effectively reduces tension on the mucosal suture line in the nasopharynx.

- If the soft palate is divided for exposure, it is repaired in three layers to minimize fistula formation
- Evaluation of the lateral ports is made. Neither port should be under tension as this increases the risk of postoperative failure. The pharyngeal flap should not be visualized in

Capra · Brigger

the oropharynx. Low lying flaps may preclude participation in velopharyngeal closure.

- Closure of the inferior donor site mucosa is performed with 3-0 vicryl suture. The superior aspect of the donor site is left to granulate.
- The previously placed cut endotracheal tubes for lateral port creation may be left in place to the level of the midoropharynx and serve as nasal stents. The author generally secures the tubes to each other extranasally and removes on postoperative day 1. If stenting is preferred to be longer duration, the stents can be secured with an anterior transseptal suture.

Postoperative Care
- Admission of patient for overnight postoperative observation
- Postoperative antibiotics are prescribed for 1 week
- Nasal stents are suctioned as necessary
- Nasal stents are removed on postoperative day 1
- Patients return for postoperative evaluation at 1 week
- Begin speech therapy 1 month postoperatively

Complications
- Postoperatively, snoring can be expected; however, persistent OSA symptoms should be addressed and may require surgical intervention
- Nasopharyngeal stenosis postoperatively also increases the risk of OSA and hyponasal speech. Persistence beyond 3 months may necessitate revision surgery.
- Persistent VPI following surgery may be improved with speech therapy. If symptoms persist beyond 3 months, revision surgery may be necessary. In some cases, this may be due to narrowing of the flap during healing or a low set flap.

Sphincter Pharyngoplasty

Indications
- Goal is to recreate a dynamic sphincter
- Coronal or circular closure patterns are most amenable to sphincter pharyngoplasty

Contraindications
Special consideration must be made in children with sleep-disordered breathing. Sphincter pharyngoplasty has a lower incidence of postoperative obstructive sleep apnea when compared to pharyngeal flap procedures.

Anesthesia Considerations
- General endotracheal anesthesia is required
- A high level of suspicion should be maintained for velo-cardio-facial syndrome and coexistent cardiac abnormalities

Preparation
- Preoperative:
- Review nasendoscopy or multiview fluoroscopy
- Intraoperative:
- Shoulder roll as necessary for neck extension
- Insert Dingman mouth gag and place into Rose position
- Posterior nasopharyngeal wall is evaluated and palpated to identify anomalous vasculature
- Rubber catheters may be placed transnasally or 2-0 silk sutures may be used to retract the soft palate to allow for better visualization of the surgical field
- The senior author routinely administer perioperative antibiotics

Procedure
For details of the procedure, see figure 3 and online supplementary video 2. 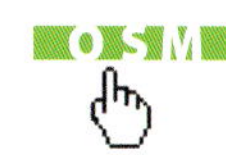
- Proposed incision lines include delineation of lateral superior-based flaps and a transverse line across the posterior pharyngeal wall at the level of velopharyngeal closure as determined

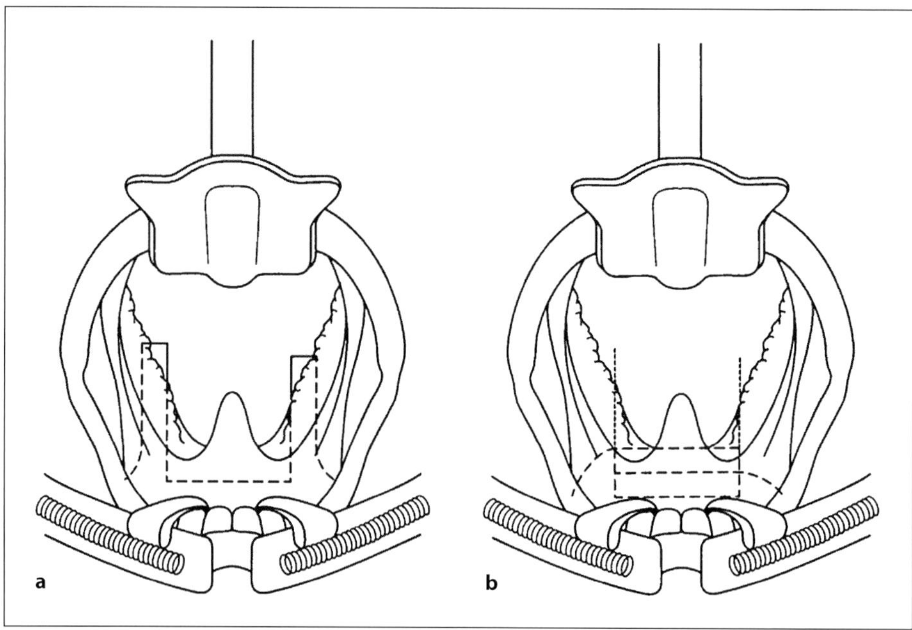

Fig. 3. a Sphincter pharyngoplasty posterior pharyngeal wall incisions. **b** Lateral flaps rotated and inset into transverse posterior pharyngeal wall incision. Reprinted with kind permission from Bluestone CD & Rosenfeld RM, Surgical Atlas of Pediatric Otolaryngology, 2002, BC Decker.

from preoperative nasendoscopy. Proposed incision lines are injected with 1% lidocaine with 1:100,000 epinephrine to aid in hemostasis of the surgical plane.

- Two superiorly based lateral flaps are created in the region of the posterior tonsillar pillars incorporating the palatopharyngeus muscle. Length is estimated by the distance required to provide adequate tissue for inset into the proposed incision at the site of velopharyngeal closure.
- A transverse incision between the medial aspect of the lateral flaps at the level of velopharyngeal closure is made to the depth of the prevertebral fascia. The mucosa is elevated superiorly to allow the lateral flaps to be inset.
- The lateral flaps are then medially rotated 90° and set into the transverse incision bed
- The flaps are secured using 3-0 vicryl sutures. They may be in tandem or parallel

to one another depending on the level of velopharyngeal closure needed.
- Donor sites are closed using 3-0 vicryl sutures

Postoperative Care
- Admission of patient for overnight postoperative observation
- Postoperative antibiotics are prescribed for 1 week
- Patients return for postoperative evaluation at 1 week
- Begin speech therapy 1 month postoperatively

Complications
- Persistent VPI following surgery may be improved with speech therapy. If symptoms persist beyond 3 months, revision surgery may be necessary. This may be due to

sphincteroplasty placement below the level of velopharyngeal closure or insufficient bulk.

- Although possible, OSA and nasopharyngeal stenosis are rare postoperative complications in sphincteroplasty

Pearls

- Identification of velopharyngeal closure patterns is essential to selecting the appropriate surgical procedure
- Speech therapy assists in patient selection, may serve as an alternative to surgery in some patients, and is essential in postoperative therapy. Postoperative resonance therapy is critical in establishing new speech patterns based on reconstructed velopharyngeal anatomy.
- Injection pharyngoplasty may be more appropriate for patients with mild VPI. Calcium hydroxyapatite has been shown to have rare extrusion, infection, resorption, or migration rates. This technique is not a contraindication for more invasive pharyngoplasty procedures in the future.
- Hypertrophic tonsils are a clinically important cause of VPI. Tonsillectomy may be curative in some cases.
- Postoperative obstructive sleep apnea and nasopharyngeal stenosis are two commonly postoperative complications. Both occur primarily in the posterior pharyngeal flap technique.
- Resolution of VPI after surgery ranges from 62 to 98% [15–24]. Research suggests no appreciable difference in outcomes between pharyngeal flaps and sphincter pharyngoplasty [see 27].
- Published revision rates range from 13 to 20% with the average being 16%. Common causes include flap placement below velopharyngeal closure, flap dehiscence, large velopharyngeal gaps, and history of craniofacial abnormalities [21, 25–28].
- Regardless of primary procedure, revision surgery may require selection of a different surgical approach
- A rolled flap technique provides a surgical alternative to injection pharyngoplasty. It includes elevating a superiorly based posterior pharyngeal wall flap and rolling it onto itself rather than inserting it to the soft palate [29].
- The Furlow procedure is another alternative for mild VPI and small velopharyngeal gaps. (Please see respective chapter.) It also provides a secondary procedure option following pharyngoplasty failure [30].

Case Presentation

A 7-year-old otherwise healthy female presented with hypernasal speech not responsive to therapy. Her mother noted that she had most difficulty with 'P' and 'S' words. The patient had no history of cleft palate or previous nasopharyngeal surgery. Of note, her younger sister has similar speech issues. The patient was witnessed to have mild snoring and daytime somnolence. Physical exam revealed a normal soft palate and uvula with 3+ tonsils. Nasendoscopy demonstrated a central velopharyngeal gap associated with air escape and good lateral wall motion. Speech pathology evaluation confirmed hypernasality most notable on vowels and pressure-sensitive consonant phonemes. Genetic testing for 22q11.2 deletion was negative. Surgical options were discussed with the patient and family, who elected to proceed with a superiorly based pharyngeal flap. Given a history suggestive of preoperative obstructive sleep apnea, a tonsillectomy was performed 6 weeks prior to the anticipated pharyngoplasty surgical date. The surgery was performed, and the postoperative course was uneventful. The otolaryngology exam showed a well-healed superiorly based pharyngeal flap. Speech therapy 3 months postoperatively showed improved speech intelligibility with minimal hypernasality.

References

1 Trost JE: Articulatory additions to the classical description of the speech of persons with cleft palate. Cleft Palate J 1981;18:193–203.
2 Brigger MT, Ashland JE, Hartnick CJ: Velopharyngeal Insufficiency; in Hartnick CJ, Boseley ME (eds): Clinical Management of Children's Voice Disorders. San Diego, Plural Publishing, 2009.
3 Witzel MA, Rich RH, Margar-Bacal F, et al: Velopharyngeal insufficiency after adenoidectomy: an 8-year review. Int J Pediatr Otorhinolaryngol 1986;11:15–20.
4 Robin NH, Shprintzen RJ: Defining the clinical spectrum of deletion 22q11.2. J Pediatr 2005;147:90–96.
5 Kummer AW, Billmire DA, Myer CM 3rd: Hypertrophic tonsils: the effect on resonance and velopharyngeal closure. Plast Reconstr Surg 1993;91:8–11.
6 Willging JP, Cotton RT: Velopharyngeal Insufficiency; in Bluestone CD, Stool SE, Alper CM (eds): Pediatric Otolaryngology, ed 4. Philadelphia, Saunders, 2003, pp 1789–1799.
7 Kamerer DB, Rood SR: The tensor tympani, stapedius, and tensor veli palatine muscles – an electromyographic study. Otolaryngology 1978;86:416–421.
8 Azzam NA, Kuehn DP: The morphology of musculus uvulae. Cleft Palate J 1977;14:78–87.
9 Shprintzen RJ, McGall GN, Skolnick ML, et al: Selective movement of the lateral aspects of the pharyngeal walls during velopharyngeal closure for speech, blowing, and whistling in normals. Cleft Palate J 1975;12:51–58.
10 Skolnick ML, McCG, Barnes M: The sphincteric mechanism of velopharyngeal closure. Cleft Palate J 1973;10:286–305.
11 Peterson-Falzone S, Trost-Cardamone J, Karnell M, et al: The Clinician's Guide to Treating Cleft Palate Speech. Mosby, St. Louis, 2005, pp 124–160.
12 Golding-Kushner KJ: Therapy techniques for cleft palate speech and related disorder; in Golding-Kushner KJ (ed): Therapy Techniques for Cleft Palate Speech and Related Disorders. Sinular, San Diego, 2001.
13 Rudnick EF, Sie KC: Velopharyngeal insufficiency: current concepts in diagnosis and management. Curr Opin Otolaryngol Head Neck Surg 2008;16:530–535.
14 Kumar S, Hedge V: Prosthodontics in velopharyngeal insufficiency. J Ind Prosthodont Soc 2007;7:12–16.
15 Argamaso RV, Levandowski GJ, Golding-Kushner KJ, et al: Treatment of asymmetric velopharyngeal insufficiency with skewed pharyngeal flap. Cleft Palate Craniofac J 1994;31:287–294.
16 Armour A, Fischbach S, Klaiman P, et al: Does velopharyngeal closure pattern affect the success of pharyngeal flap pharyngoplasty? Plast Reconstr Surg 2005;115:45–52, discussion 53.
17 Chegar BE, Shprintzen RJ, Curtis MS, et al: Pharyngeal flap and obstructive apnea: maximizing speech outcome while limiting complications. Arch Facial Plast Surg 2007;9:252–259.
18 de Serres LM, Deleyiannis FW, Eblen LE, et al: Results with sphincter pharyngoplasty and pharyngeal flap. Int J Pediatr Otorhinolaryngol 1999;48:17–25.
19 Lendrum J, Dhar BK: The Orticochea dynamic pharyngoplasty. Br J Plast Surg 1984;37:160–168.
20 Meek MF, Coert JH, Hofer SO, et al: Short-term and long-term results of speech improvement after surgery for velopharyngeal insufficiency with pharyngeal flaps in patients younger and older than 6 years old: 10-year experience. Ann Plast Surg 2003;50:13–17.
21 Pryor LS, Lehman J, Parker MG, et al: Outcomes in pharyngoplasty: a 10-year experience. Cleft Palate Craniofac J 2006; 43:222–225.
22 Seagle MB, Mazaheri MK, Dixon-Wood VL, et al: Evaluation and treatment of velopharyngeal insufficiency: the University of Florida experience. Ann Plast Surg 2002;48:464–470.
23 Sie KC, Chen EY: Management of velopharyngeal insufficiency: development of a protocol and modifications of sphincter pharyngoplasty. Facial Plast Surg 2007;23:128–139.
24 Sie KC, Tampakopoulou DA, de Serres LM, et al: Sphincter pharyngoplasty: speech outcome and complications. Laryngoscope 1998;108:1211–1217.
25 Witt PD, Myckatyn T, Marssh JL: Salvaging the failed pharyngoplasty: intervention outcome. Cleft Palate Craniofac J 1998;35:447–453.
26 Sloan GM: Posterior pharyngeal flap and sphincter pharyngoplasty: the state of the art. Cleft Palate Craniofac J 2000;37:112–122.
27 Abyholm F, D'Antonio L, Davidson Ward SL, et al: Pharyngeal flap and sphincterplasty for velopharyngeal insufficiency have equal outcome at 1 year postoperatively: results of a randomized trial. Cleft Palate Craniofac J 2005;42:501–511.
28 Losken A, Williams JK, Burstein FD, et al: An outcome evaluation of sphincter pharyngoplasty for the management of velopharyngeal insufficiency. Plast Reconstr Surg 2003;112:1755–1761.
29 Brigger MT, Ashland JE, Hartnick CJ: Injection pharyngoplasty with calcium hydroxylapatite for velopharyngeal insufficiency: patient selection and technique. Arch Otolaryngol Head Neck Surg 2010;136:666–670.
30 D'Antonio LL: Correction of velopharyngeal insufficiency using the Furlow double-opposing Z-plasty. West J Med 1997;167:101–102.

Matthew T. Brigger, MD, MPH, LCDR MC USN
Naval Medical Center San Diego
Department of Otolaryngology, Head and Neck Surgery
34800 Bob Wilson Drive
San Diego, CA 92134 (USA)
E-Mail matthew.brigger@med.navy.mil

Hartnick CJ, Hansen MC, Gallagher TQ (eds): Pediatric Airway Surgery. Adv Otorhinolaryngol. Basel, Karger, 2012, vol 73, pp 145–148

Double-Reversing Z-Plasty (Furlow Palatoplasty)

Mark Boseley · Scott E. Bevans

Otolaryngology – Head and Neck Surgery, Madigan Army Medical Center, MCHJ-CLS-E, Tacoma, Wash., USA

Abstract

Dr. Leonard Furlow first described the double-reversing z-plasty technique for cleft soft palate repair in 1978. This approach allows for repair of an overt or submucous cleft palate, but just as an importantly, provides additional length to the palate and also realigns the palatal musculature. The Furlow palatoplasty (the name by which the procedure is commonly referred) has therefore been instrumental in the treatment of velopharyngeal insufficiency. The primary aims of this chapter are to provide the clinician with the indications for when to consider utilizing the Furlow palatoplasty and to give a stepwise description of how to perform the procedure.

Dr. Leonard Furlow first described the double-reversing Z-plasty technique for overt and soft palate cleft repair in 1978. This approach was designed to not only provide separation of the nasal and oral cavities, but also to increase palate length and to create an intact muscular sling. The Z-plasty allows for lengthening of the palatal tissues while closing the midline defect.

The key muscles involved in velopharyngeal closure are the tensor veli palatini, the musculus uvulae and the levator veli palatini. These muscles insert onto the posterior side of the soft palate in overt cleft palate patients. The levator veli palatini lies in a sagittal orientation in submucous cleft palate patients [1]. When considering the type of repair, it is important that these muscles are reoriented into a transverse position in order to provide for optimal velopharyngeal closure.

Currently, the double-reversing z-plasty repair is primarily used for isolated soft palate and submucous clefts. When comparing this technique with others, it is important to look at objective measurements of palatal function (i.e. velopharyngeal competence), in addition to achievement of closure of the defect. Perhaps the largest prospective study to date (376 children) comparing another common technique for cleft palate repair (von Langenbeck) to the Furlow palatoplasty, revealed that speech outcomes were better in the Furlow palatoplasty group [2]. A second study examined the role of the double-reversing z-plasty in children with velo-cardio-facial syndrome who had a submucous cleft palate as part of their syndrome. These authors found that the Furlow technique is best utilized when the palate was noted to be mobile. Otherwise, they felt that a posterior pharyngeal flap gave the best speech results in patients with a submucous cleft palate [3].

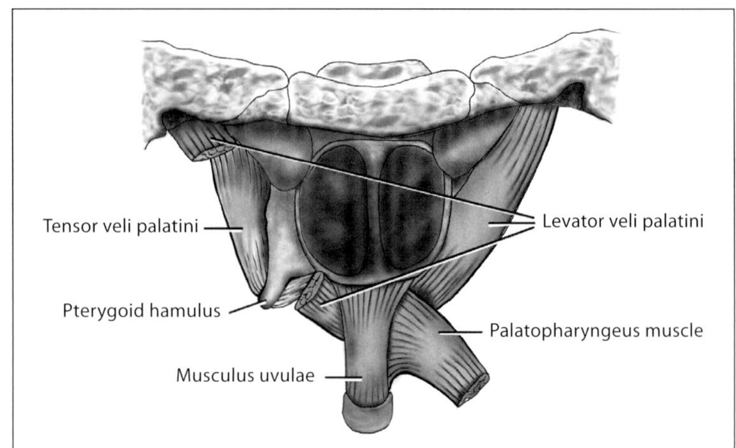

Fig. 1. Palatal muscles.

The senior author utilizes the Furlow palatoplasty in his practice for overt soft palate defects that are less than 1 cm in length. This technique is also their primary choice to repair submucous cleft palates in children with velopharyngeal insufficiencies that have failed an attempt at speech therapy. Finally, although the surgical planes can be quite difficult to ascertain, the senior author uses this flap in children who have already had a primary repair of their cleft palate but appear to have nasal air escape secondary to having a shortened soft palate. It is the author's opinion that the sphincter pharyngoplasty procedure is a better option for children with poor velopharyngeal closure due to decreased lateral wall motion on nasoendoscopy. Finally, injection palatoplasty should be considered for small gaps in the velopharyngeal port, often after the child has had a prior procedure performed for their VPI.

Relevant Anatomy

For relevant anatomy, see figure 1.

Indications

- Isolated cleft soft palate
- Submucous cleft palate
- Persistent velopharyngeal insufficiency due to a shortened soft palate following primary repair

Contraindications

Wide soft palate defects.

Anesthesia Considerations

Midline endotracheal tube – oral Rae or armored tube is preferred to prevent 'kinking' of the tube during the course of the procedure.

Intraoperative Preparation

- Dingman mouth retractor is preferred in order to maximize visualization
- Generous shoulder roll for neck extension if surgeon seated for the procedure
- Mark proposed Z-plasty incisions with either gentian violet or a surgical marker
- Local injection with lidocaine with 1:100,000 epinephrine along proposed incision lines

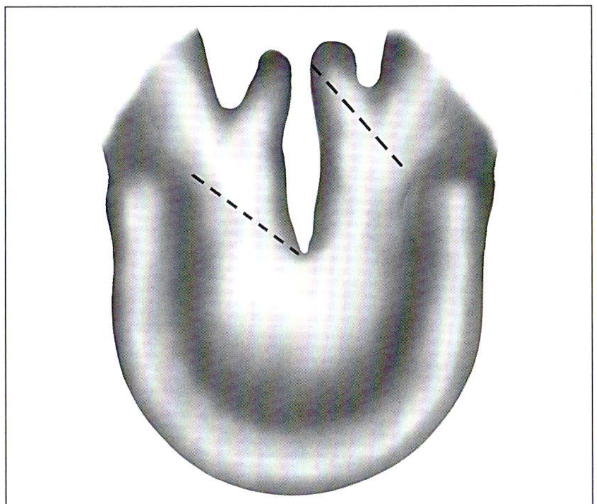

Fig. 2. First cuts.

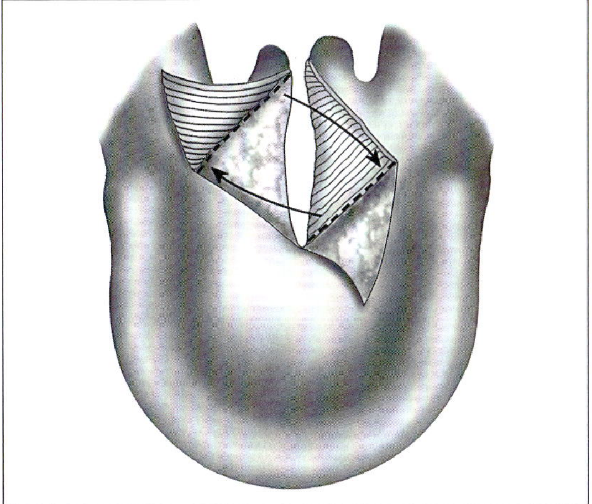

Fig. 3. Second cuts.

Procedure

- An incision is made with a 15 blade through the mucosa on the patient's right side, from the posterior edge of the cleft laterally toward the hamulus to create an anterior-based mucosal flap (online suppl. video 1)
- This mucosal flap can be raised with a combination of sharp and blunt dissection. The 60° Potts scissors, Langenbeck elevator and the Pennington elevator work well for this purpose. Care must be taken to minimize trauma to this flap, since it can be quite thin (fig. 2).
- A second incision is then made with a 15 blade through the mucosa and the levator musculature on the patient's left side, from the hard-soft palate junction laterally toward the hamulus to create a posterior-based myomucosal flap (fig. 2)
- The myomucosal flap can then be raised in a posterior direction, taking care not to disrupt the nasopharyngeal mucosa on the posterior surface (fig. 2, 3)
- If performed for a submucous cleft palate, the author will wait until all of the flaps are elevated prior to making the midline incision in order to provide countertraction while elevating the flaps

- If performed for an overt cleft palate, the midline mucosal palate incision is best accomplished with a 60° angled beaver blade
- Angled scissors are then used to make the opposing Z-plasty incisions. On the patient's right side, this incision is through the levator muscle and nasopharyngeal mucosa. On the patient's left side, this incision is through the nasopharyngeal mucosa only (fig. 3). 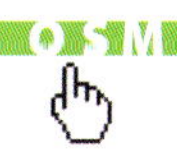
- The nasal side z-plasty is now closed by first suturing the right-sided posterior-based myomucosal flap to the cut surface of the nasopharyngeal mucosa on the left side with 3-0 or 4-0 chromic suture (fig. 4)
- The anterior-based left-sided nasopharyngeal mucosal flap is then inset by suturing it to the anterior surface of levator muscle described in the above step, and to the cut under surface of the right-sided oral mucosal flap with 3-0 or 4-0 chromic suture (fig. 4)
- The oral side z-plasty is then closed by first suturing the left-sided posterior-based oral mucosal and levator muscle flap to the cut surface of the oral mucosa on the right side with 4-0 vicryl suture (fig. 5)
- Finally, the right-sided anterior-based oral mucosal flap is sutured into place with 4-0 vicryl

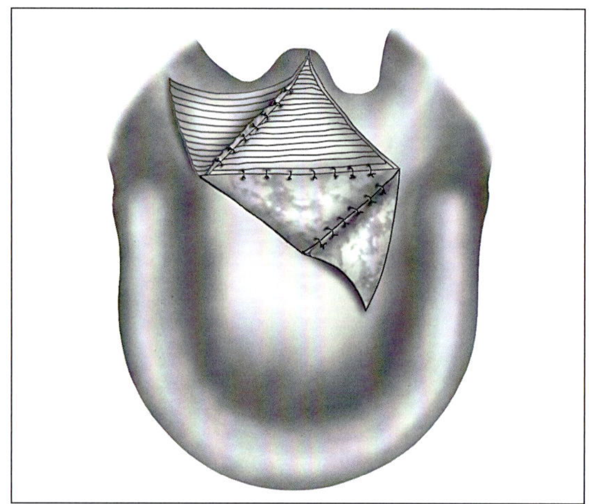

Fig. 4. First layer closure.

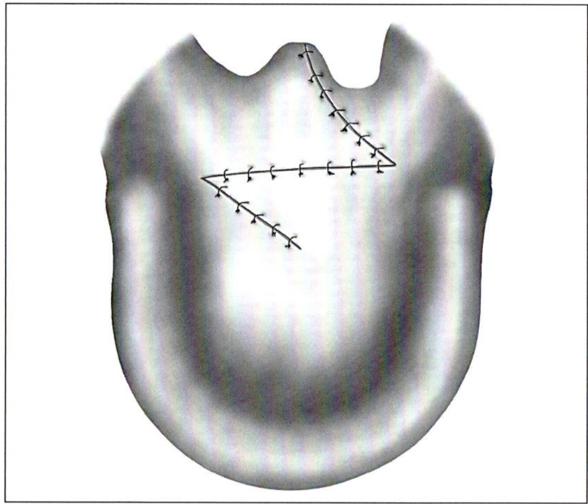

Fig. 5. Complete closure.

suture. This flap covers the nasopharyngeal mucosal flap (fig. 5).

Postoperative Care

- Care must be taken to prevent trauma to the repair. This might involve use of arm restraints during the postoperative period if the child has a propensity to put his/her fingers in the mouth. Also, the use of 'sippy' cups and straws should be avoided for approximately 3 weeks after surgery.
- Solid foods should be of a pureed consistency for 3 weeks following surgery
- Antibiotics should be used for 5–7 days following surgery

Surgical Pearls

- Adequate hemostasis is vital in order to properly identify the surgical planes of dissection
- The anterior-based mucosal flap can be quite delicate. The senior author has found that it is important to keep some minor salivary gland tissue on the posterior surface of this flap in order for it to withstand more tension when closing the mucosal layer.
- When closing the mucosal layer, the senior author has found that there can be significant tension on the flaps. It can sometimes require some 'trial and error' when placing the first sutures. The key is to inset the flaps with the least amount of tension possible.

References

1 Chiu LL, Sie K: Sphincter pharyngoplasty for management of velopharyngeal insufficiency. Oper Techniques Otolaryngol Head Neck Surg 2009;20: 263–267.

2 Williams WN, Seagle MB, Pegoraro-Krook MI, et al: Prospective clinical trial comparing outcome measures between Furlow and von Langenbeck palatoplasties for UCLP. Ann Plast Surg 2011;66:154–163.

3 Rottgers SA, Ford M, Cray J, et al: An algorithm for application of Furlow palatoplasty to the treatment of velocardiofacial syndrome-associated velopharyngeal insufficiency. Ann Plast Surg 2011;66:479–484.

Mark Boseley, MD, LTC
Madigan Army Medical Center
MCHJ-CLS-E, BLDG 9048, Jackson Ave.
Tacoma, WA 98431-1110 (USA)
E-Mail mark.boseley@us.army.mil

Hartnick CJ, Hansen MC, Gallagher TQ (eds): Pediatric Airway Surgery. Adv Otorhinolaryngol. Basel, Karger, 2012, vol 73, pp 149–152

Pediatric Sialendoscopy

Jean M. Bruch · Jennifer Setlur

Department of Otolaryngology, Massachusetts Eye & Ear Infirmary, Boston, Mass., USA

Abstract

Sialendoscopy was introduced in the early 1990s as a minimally invasive alternative to standard methods for diagnosis and treatment of inflammatory and obstructive salivary gland disease. The technique was pioneered in adults; however, advances in instrumentation have allowed this to be adapted to the smaller salivary ductal anatomy found in the pediatric population. In this chapter, the technique of sialendoscopy for parotid and submandibular glands is described.

Sialendoscopy was introduced in the early 1990s as a minimally invasive alternative to standard methods for diagnosis and treatment of inflammatory and obstructive salivary gland disease. The technique was pioneered in adults; however, advances in instrumentation have allowed this to be adapted to the smaller salivary ductal anatomy found in the pediatric population. Although salivary gland disease is less common in children, comprising approximately 10% of all cases [1], it represents a source of significant morbidity in those affected, with mumps and juvenile recurrent parotitis (JRP) being the two most common etiologies [2]. Sialolithiasis is seen much more frequently in adults; however, it does occur in children. Salivary stones in the pediatric population overall are found to be smaller and present with shorter duration of symptoms [3–5].

Prior to the introduction of endoscopy, treatment of salivary gland disease was limited to conservative methods (antibiotics, sialagogues, massage, warm compresses, maintenance of hydration) or more aggressive surgical procedures (duct ligation, tympanic neurectomy, intra-oral duct lithotomy, gland excision), all of which are associated with a variety of drawbacks and risks [2]. Endoscopy allows direct visualization of the ductal system with more accurate identification and localization of pathology such as stones, strictures, mucous plugging, and anatomic abnormalities. Traditional diagnostic modalities including plain radiographs, CT, ultrasound, sialography, and MR pose limitations with respect to radiation exposure, poor resolution of small or radiolucent stones, and difficulty distinguishing between stones and stenoses [6, 7]. Use of these methods in the pediatric population can also prove to be more challenging than with adults.

Therapeutic intervention with endoscopy is possible in many cases by means of stone extraction, dilatation of stenotic segments, ductal lavage with irrigation of debris from tertiary ducts (such as fibrinous exudate, mucous plugs, and inflammatory mediators) and instillation of anti-inflammatory medications. In addition, this can be performed at the same time as the diagnostic procedure. In the case of JRP, endoscopic findings typically include a white avascular appearance of the duct lumen with stenotic segments [8]. Dilatation (using the endoscope itself, hydrostatic pressure from the irrigant, and instruments passed through the working channel of the endoscope) followed by instillation of corticosteroid can result in substantial improvement in symptoms [1, 9, 10]. Stone extraction for lithiasis can be achieved via basket extraction through the duct orifice with or without adjunctive stone fragmentation using laser or lithotripsy [7, 11]. A combined approach using endoscopic localization in conjunction with targeted extra-oral removal can also be used for large stones. By breaking the cycle of obstruction and inflammation, an otherwise chronically involved gland may be salvaged and remain functional and symptom free [12].

In this chapter, the technique of sialendoscopy for parotid and submandibular glands is described. Investment in specialized equipment is necessary, including semi-rigid miniature endoscopes and accessories for stone removal and duct 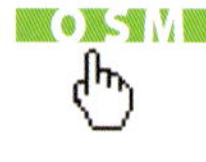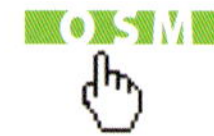 dilatation. The endoscopes are adaptable to standard camera and video tower setups commonly used for endoscopic sinus surgery.

Indications

- Chronic and acute inflammatory or obstructive conditions of the parotid and submandibular glands including:
- Sialolithiasis (stones measuring 3–5 mm in greatest dimension for parotid cases or 4–7 mm in submandibular cases)
- JRP and Sjogren's syndrome
- Anatomic ductal strictures, congenital or acquired

Contraindications

- Active bacterial infection, which may increase risk of duct perforation

- Stones larger than 5–7 mm may require fragmentation with either a holmium laser or lithotripsy before endoscopic extraction. Very large stones usually necessitate the use of a combined technique for stone removal.

Preoperative Preparation and Anesthetic Considerations

- Standard oral or nasal endotracheal intubation
- Intravenous dexamethasone (0.5 mg/kg, maximum dose of 10 mg)
- Intraoperative antibiotics, 1 dose i.v. at start of procedure (dosed per body weight) with additional doses at the discretion of surgeon

Equipment

- Sialendoscopes: 0.8-, 1.1-, and 1.6-mm outer diameter (see online suppl. video 1)
- 0.8-mm scope has irrigation channel only with no working channel for passage of instruments
- Larger scopes (1.1 and 1.6 mm) accommodate passage of guidewire, microdrill, wire basket, and laser fiber through working channel
- A 1.6-mm scope is available, which will allow use of grasping and biopsy forceps; however, it may be too large for pediatric applications
- Camera and video tower
- Pixel density: due to the small size of the scope, image quality is limited by the size and number of fiber-optic bundles. High-quality endoscopes and camera equipment will maximize image resolution.
- Irrigation tubing and 5- or 10-ml syringe or i.v. bag
- Bite block or Medesey mouth gag
- Salivary probes/dilators
Accessory instruments: guide wire, dilators, microdrill, wire extraction baskets, balloons,

and stents. (Note that balloons are not currently available for use in the US pending FDA approval.)

Surgical Procedure

- The salivary gland papilla (parotid or submandibular) is identified and cannulated with salivary duct probes and papilla dilator
- Positioning of bite blocks, mouth gag, or retractors as needed to facilitate access to papilla
- Papilla is serially dilated until it can accommodate insertion of endoscope
- Endoscope is atraumatically advanced within the main duct under direct vision with continuous saline irrigation; endoscope can then be advanced into secondary and tertiary branches
- Pathology is noted and addressed:
- Stones: extraction through oral cavity with wire basket or grasping forceps may require papillotomy. Advanced techniques utilizing combined endoscopic/external approach and fragmentation with microdrill, laser, lithotripsy
- Strictures: dilatation using bougies over guide wire, endoscope tip, microdrill, balloon catheter, hydrostatic pressure from irrigation
- Mucous plugging, fibrinous exudates, plaques: lavage with saline, 60 ml per gland
- Careful exploration of the ductal system following treatment of pathology to assess for injury
- Stenting of the duct may be required for significant stenosis or injury
- Instillation of corticosteroid (Kenalog 40, hydrocortisone 100 mg, or methylprednisolone 150 mg) into the duct can be done through the endoscope irrigation or working channel

Postoperative Care

- Postoperative observation in monitored setting with same day discharge when patient meets standard criteria
- Routine postoperative antibiotics are not administered
- Pain control as needed
- This procedure is not typically painful. The patient may experience uncomfortable gland swelling secondary to volume of irrigation, which typically resolves with massage over 24 h.
- Maintain hydration status and salivary flow with sialagogues
- Pressure dressing if combined extra-oral approach is used for parotid gland
- No significant limitation of activities is required

Pearls

- Use of operative loupes facilitates identification of the duct orifice
- Atraumatic insertion and advancement of endoscope is critical to avoid inadvertent duct perforation or injury leading to stenosis
- Continuous gentle irrigation prevents duct collapse and poor visualization
- Papillotomy may be required to deliver stone/basket through narrow orifice
- Avoid papillotomy in early stages of procedure, as this can interfere with visualization due to loss of irrigant and duct collapse
- Stenting of the duct may be necessary in certain cases such as dilatation of a tight stenosis
- Irrigation of the parotid may cause swelling in the pharynx/deep portion of gland. Be careful to assess for airway compromise if bilateral glands are treated.

References

1 Konstantinidis I, Dhatziavramidis A, Tsakiropoulou E, Malliari H, Constantinidis J: Pediatric sialendoscopy under local anesthesia: limitations and potentials. Int J Pediatr Otorhinolaryngol 2011;75:245–249.

2 Katz P, Hartl DM, Guerre A: Treatment of juvenile recurrent parotitis. Otolaryngol Clin North Am 2009;42:1087–1091.

3 Chung MK, Jeong HS, Ko MH, Cho HJ, Rue NG, Cho DY, Son Y, Baek C: Pediatric sialolithiasis: what is different from adult sialolithiasis? Int J Pediatr Otorhinolaryngol 2007;71:787–791.

4 Faure F, Querin S, Dulguerov P, Froehlich P, Dissant F, Marchal F: Pediatric salivary gland obstructive swelling: sialendoscopic approach. Laryngoscope 2007;117:1364–1367.

5 Nahlieli O, Eliav E, Hasson O, Zagury A, Baruchin AM: Pediatric sialolithiasis. Oral Surg Oral Med Oral Pathol Oral Radiol Endod 2000;90:709–712.

6 Martins-Carvalho C, Plouin-Gaudon I, Quenin S, Lesniak J, Froehlich P, Marchal F: Pediatric sialendoscopy: a 5-year experience at a single institution. Arch Otolaryngol Head Neck Surg 2010;136:33–36.

7 Faure F, Froehlich P, Marchal F: Paediatric sialendoscopy. Curr Opin Otolaryngol Head Neck Surg 2008;16:60–63.

8 Nahlieli O, Sacham R, Shlesinger M, Eliav E: Juvenile recurrent parotitis: a new method of diagnosis and treatment. Pediatrics 2004;114:9–12.

9 Sacham R, Droma EB, London D, Bar T, Nahlieli O: Long term experience with endoscopic diagnosis and treatment of juvenile recurrent parotitis. J Oral Maxilofac Surg 2009;67:162–167.

10 Quenin S, Plouin-Gaudon I, Marchal F, Froelich P, Disant F, Faure F: Juvenile recurrent parotitis. Arch Otolaryngol Head Neck Surg 2008;134:715–719.

11 McJunkin J, Milov S, Jeyakumar A: Lithotripsy for refractory pediatric sialolithiasis. Laryngoscope 2009;119:298–299.

12 Jabbour N, Tibesar R, Lander T, Sidman J: Sialendoscopy in children. Int J Pediatr Otorhinolaryngol 2010;74:347–350.

Jean M. Bruch, DMD, MD
Massachusetts Eye and Ear Infirmary, Department of Otolaryngology
243 Charles St
Boston, MA 02114 (USA)
E-Mail jean_bruch@meei.harvard.edu

Author Index